Diagnostic Imaging of Intestinal Ischemia and Infarction

Guest Editor

Stefania Romano, MD

RADIOLOGIC
CLINICS OF NORTH AMERICA

www.radiologic.theclinics.com

September 2008 • Volume 46 • Number 5

SAUNDERS an imprint of ELSEVIER, Inc.

W.B. SAUNDERS COMPANY
A Division of Elsevier Inc.

1600 John F. Kennedy Boulevard • Suite 1800 • Philadelphia, Pennsylvania 19103-2899

http://www.theclinics.com

RADIOLOGIC CLINICS OF NORTH AMERICA Volume 46, Number 5
September 2008 ISSN 0033-8389, ISBN 13: 978-1-4160-6348-3, ISBN 10: 1-4160-6348-X

Editor: Barton Dudlick

Radiologic Clinics of North America (ISSN 0033-8389) is published bimonthly in January, March, May, July, September, and November by Elsevier Inc., 360 Park Avenue South, New York, NY 10010-1710. Business and Editorial Offices: 1600 John F. Kennedy Boulevard., Suite 1800, Philadelphia, PA 19103-2899. Customer Service Office: 6277 Sea Harbor Drive, Orlando, FL 32887-4800. Periodicals postage paid at New York, NY and additional mailing offices. Subscription prices are USD 290 per year for US individuals, USD 431 per year for US institutions, USD 142 per year for US students and residents, USD 339 per year for Canadian individuals, USD 530 per year for Canadian institutions, USD 394 per year for international individuals, USD 530 per year for international institutions, and USD 192 per year for Canadian and foreign students/residents. To receive student and resident rate, orders must be accompanied by name of affiliated institution, date of term and the signature of program/residency coordinatior on institution letterhead. Orders will be billed at individual rate until proof of status is received. Foreign air speed delivery is included in all *Clinics* subscription prices. All prices are subject to change without notice. **POSTMASTER:** Send address changes to *Radiologic Clinics of North America*, Elsevier Journals Customer Service, 6277 Sea Harbor Drive, Orlando, FL 32887-4800. **Customer Service: 1-800-654-2452 (US). From outside of the United States, call (+1) 407-563-6020. Fax: 407-363-9661. E-mail: JournalsCustomerService-usa@elsevier.com.**

Reprints. For copies of 100 or more of articles in this publication, please contact the Commercial Reprints Department, Elsevier Inc., 360 Park Avenue South, New York, New York 10010-1710. Tel.: (+1) 212-633-3812; Fax: (+1) 212-462-1935; E-mail: reprints@elsevier.com.

Radiologic Clinics of North America also published in Greek Paschalidis Medical Publications, Athens, Greece.

Radiologic Clinics of North America is covered in *MEDLINE/PubMed (Index Medicus), EMBASE/Excerpta Medica, Current Contents/Life Sciences, Current Contents/Clinical Medicine, RSNA Index to Imaging Literature, BIOSIS, Science Citation Index,* and *ISI/BIOMED*.

Printed in the United States of America.

Contributors

GUEST EDITOR

STEFANIA ROMANO, MD
Department of Diagnostic Imaging, Section
of General and Emergency Radiology,
"A. Cardarelli" Hospital, Naples, Italy

AUTHORS

MARIANO FORTUNATO ARMELLINO, MD
Department of General and Emergency Surgery
with Polyspecialistic Observation, "A. Cardarelli"
Hospital, Naples, Italy

SOPHIE AUFORT, MD
Department of Imaging, CHU Montpellier, Hospital
St Eloi, Montpellier, France

GIOVANNI BARTONE, MD
Department of General and Emergency Surgery,
"A. Cardarelli" Hospital, Naples, Italy

JONATHAN W. BERLIN, MD
Department of Radiology, Evanston Northwestern
Healthcare, Northwestern University Medical
School, Evanston, Illinois

CHERI L. CANON, MD
Associate Professor, Vice Chair for Education,
Director of Radiology Residency Program,
Chief of GI Section, Department of Radiology,
University of Alabama at Birmingham,
Birmingham, Alabama

MAURIZIO CASTRICONI, MD
Department of General and Emergency Surgery,
"A. Cardarelli" Hospital, Naples, Italy

ERIC DELABROUSSE, MD
Department of Imaging, CHU Besançon,
Besançon, France

FERNANDA CURROS DOYON, MD
Department of Imaging, CHU Montpellier,
Hospital Lapeyronie, Montpellier, France

RICHARD M. GORE, MD
Department of Radiology, Evanston Northwestern
Healthcare, Northwestern University Medical
School, Evanston, Illinois

MARINE DEVAUX HOQUET, MD
Department of Imaging, CHU Montpellier, Hospital
Lapeyronie, Montpellier, France

MARK E. LOCKHART, MD, MPH
Associate Professor, Associate Director of
Medical Student Education, Director of Abdominal
Imaging Fellowship Program, Department of
Radiology, University of Alabama at Birmingham,
Birmingham, Alabama

WALTER E. LONGO, MD, FACS, FASCRS
Professor of Surgery, Director of Surgical
Education, Yale University School of Medicine,
Department of Surgery; and Chief, Section of
Gastrointestinal Surgery, Yale New Haven
Hospital, New Haven, Connecticut

MAURO NATALE DOMENICO MAGLIO, MD
Department of General and Emergency Surgery,
"A. Cardarelli" Hospital, Naples, Italy

FRANCO MAGLIONE, MD
Department of Diagnostic Imaging, Section
of Vascular and Interventional Radiology,
"A. Cardarelli" Hospital, Naples, Italy

UDAY K. MEHTA, MD
Department of Radiology, Evanston Northwestern
Healthcare, Northwestern University Medical
School, Evanston, Illinois

SAMUEL MERIGEAUD, MD
Department of Imaging, CHU Montpellier,
Hospital Lapeyronie, Montpellier, France

FRANK H. MILLER, MD
Department of Radiology, Northwestern Memorial
Hospital, Northwestern University Medical School,
Chicago, Illinois

GERALDINE M. NEWMARK, MD
Department of Radiology, Evanston Northwestern
Healthcare, Northwestern University Medical
School, Evanston, Illinois

RAFFAELLA NIOLA, MD
Department of Diagnostic Imaging, Section
of Vascular and Interventional Radiology,
"A. Cardarelli" Hospital, Naples, Italy

FLAVIO PATERNO, MD
Surgical Resident, General Surgery, Yale
University School of Medicine, Department
of Surgery, New Haven, Connecticut

LUIGIA ROMANO, MD
Department of Diagnostic Imaging, Section
of General and Emergency Radiology,
"A. Cardarelli" Hospital, Naples, Italy

STEFANIA ROMANO, MD
Department of Diagnostic Imaging, Section
of General and Emergency Radiology,
"A. Cardarelli" Hospital, Naples, Italy

BEATRICE ULLOA SEVERINO, MD
Department of General and Emergency Surgery,
"A. Cardarelli" Hospital, Naples, Italy

P. TAOUREL, MD, PhD
Department of Imaging, CHU Montpellier,
Hospital Lapeyronie, Montpellier, France

KIRAN H. THAKRAR, MD
Department of Radiology, Evanston Northwestern
Healthcare, Northwestern University Medical
School, Evanston, Illinois

HEIDI UMPHREY, MD
Resident, Department of Radiology,
University of Alabama at Birmingham,
Birmingham, Alabama

VAHID YAGHMAI, MD
Department of Radiology, Northwestern
Memorial Hospital, Northwestern University
Medical School, Chicago, Illinois

Contents

> Intestinal ischemia and infarction are a heterogeneous group of diseases that have as their unifying theme hypoxia of the small bowel or colon. The incidence of bowel ischemia and infarction is on the rise for several reasons: the aging of the population, the ability of intensive care units to salvage critically ill patients, and heightened clinical awareness of these disorders. Improvements in diagnostic imaging techniques have greatly contributed to the earlier diagnosis of intestinal ischemia, which can have a positive influence on patient outcomes. In this article, role of radiology in the detection, differential diagnosis, and management of patients who have intestinal ischemia and infarction is discussed.

> Intestinal ischemia includes all the conditions in which the blood supply to the gastrointestinal tract is not adequate to its metabolic demand. Several ischemic intestinal disorders differ in clinical presentation (acute versus chronic), etiology (occlusive versus nonocclusive), pathophysiology (arterial or venous), severity (mucosal versus transmural necrosis), and location (small bowel versus large bowel). Atherosclerosis, thromboembolic disease, hypoperfusion states, and hypercoagulable disorders are the most common causes. Reperfusion, oxygen-derived free radicals, and eicosanoids contribute to the pathogenesis of bowel injury and the systemic response that occur after ischemia. The diagnosis and treatment of intestinal ischemia are still challenging despite the advances of radiology, intensive care, and surgery. This article reviews the latest data about etiology and pathophysiology of bowel ischemia to explain the bases of diagnosis and treatment of this condition.

> Despite advances made in the diagnostic and therapeutic field, acute intestinal ischemia remains a highly lethal condition. This is related to the variability of symptoms and the absence of typical laboratory alterations in early stage.

venous gas, portal venous gas, or absence of bowel wall enhancement. Less specific imaging findings include small bowel wall thickening, mesenteric stranding, and mesenteric fluid. Further complicating the issue, several small intestinal disease processes may mimic ischemia both clinically and radiographically. These alternate diagnoses include infectious, inflammatory, and infiltrative processes.

Radiologic Clinics of North America

THE CLINICS ARE NOW AVAILABLE ONLINE!

Access your subscription at:
www.theclinics.com

GOAL STATEMENT
The goal of the *Radiologic Clinics of North America* is to keep practicing radiologists and radiology residents up to date with current clinical practice in radiology by providing timely articles reviewing the state of the art in patient care.

ACCREDITATION
The *Radiologic Clinics of North America* is planned and implemented in accordance with the Essential Areas and Policies of the Accreditation Council for Continuing Medical Education (ACCME) through the joint sponsorship of the University of Virginia School of Medicine and Elsevier. The University of Virginia School of Medicine is accredited by the ACCME to provide continuing medical education for physicians.

The University of Virginia School of Medicine designates this educational activity for a maximum of 15 *AMA PRA Category 1 Credits*™. Physicians should only claim credit commensurate with the extent of their participation in the activity.

The American Medical Association has determined that physicians not licensed in the US who participate in this CME activity are eligible for 15 *AMA PRA Category 1 Credits*™.

Credit can be earned by reading the text material, taking the CME examination online at http://www.theclinics.com/home/cme, and completing the evaluation. After taking the test, you will be required to review any and all incorrect answers. Following completion of the test and evaluation, your credit will be awarded and you may print your certificate.

FACULTY DISCLOSURE/CONFLICT OF INTEREST
The University of Virginia School of Medicine, as an ACCME accredited provider, endorses and strives to comply with the Accreditation Council for Continuing Medical Education (ACCME) Standards of Commercial Support, Commonwealth of Virginia statutes, University of Virginia policies and procedures, and associated federal and private regulations and guidelines on the need for disclosure and monitoring of proprietary and financial interests that may affect the scientific integrity and balance of content delivered in continuing medical education activities under our auspices.

The University of Virginia School of Medicine requires that all CME activities accredited through this institution be developed independently and be scientifically rigorous, balanced and objective in the presentation/discussion of its content, theories and practices.

All authors/editors participating in an accredited CME activity are expected to disclose to the readers relevant financial relationships with commercial entities occurring within the past 12 months (such as grants or research support, employee, consultant, stock holder, member of speakers bureau, etc.). The University of Virginia School of Medicine will employ appropriate mechanisms to resolve potential conflicts of interest to maintain the standards of fair and balanced education to the reader. Questions about specific strategies can be directed to the Office of Continuing Medical Education, University of Virginia School of Medicine, Charlottesville, Virginia.

The faculty and staff of the University of Virginia Office of Continuing Medical Education have no financial affiliations to disclose.

The authors/editors listed below have identified no financial or professional relationships for themselves or their spouse/partner:
Mariano Fortunato Armellino, MD; Sophie Aufort, MD; Giovanni Bartone, MD; Cheri L. Canon, MD; Maruizio Castriconi, MD; Eric Delabrousse, MD; Fernando Curros Doyon, MD; Barton Dudlick (Acquisitions Editor); Richard M. Gore, MD; Marine Devaux Hoquet, MD; Theodore E. Keats, MD (Test Author); Mark E. Lockhart, MD, MPH; Walter E. Longo, MD, FACS, FASCRS; Maruo Natale Domenico Maglio, MD; Franco Maglione, MD; Uday K. Mehta, MD; Samuel Merigeaud, MD; Frank H. Miller, MD; Geraldine M. Newmark, MD; Raffaella Niola MD; Flavio Paterno, MD; Luigia Romano, MD; Stefania Romano, MD (Guest Editor); Beatrice Ulloa Severino, MD; Patrice Taourel, MD, PhD; Kiran H. Thakrar, MD; and Vahid Yaghmai, MD.

The authors/editors listed below have identified the following financial or professional relationships for themselves or their spouse/partner:
Jonathan W. Berlin, MD owns stock and serves on the Advisory Board for Nuance Communications.
Heidi Umphrey, MD owns stock in Medical Properties and Celgene.

Disclosure of Discussion of Non-FDA Approved Uses for Pharmaceutical and/or Medical Devices
The University of Virginia School of Medicine, as an ACCME provider, requires that all faculty presenters identify and disclose any off-label uses for pharmaceutical and medical device products. The University of Virginia School of Medicine recommends that each physician fully review all the available data on new products or procedures prior to clinical use.

TO ENROLL
To enroll in the Radiologic Clinics of North America Continuing Medical Education program, call customer service at 1-800-654-2452 or sign up online at http://www.theclinics.com/home/cme. The CME program is available to subscribers for an additional annual fee USD 205.

Preface

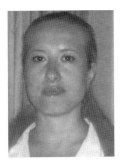

Stefania Romano, MD
Guest Editor

In the last few years, emergency radiology has gained a prominent role in the management of acute patients thanks to the modern and advanced imaging technologies that help radiologists to correctly interpret examination findings, giving important support to the referring clinicians and surgeons for a prompt and appropriate therapy. The acute abdomen represents one of the most common nontraumatic body emergencies. Intestinal ischemia is a condition that requires extreme attention because potentially lethal complications from infarction can be avoided if a prompt and appropriate diagnosis is effected.

In 2000, my mentor gave me the task of preparing a paper on intestinal infarctions of the small bowel for the final examination of my residency program. Reading the bibliographic material he had collected and becoming aware of the many obscure points under his guidance, I began to develop a "feeling" for vascular disease affecting the intestine that has grown since then. In 2001 when I entered radiology practice at my institution, which is one of the largest emergency hospitals in Italy, I had the chance to further my interest in diagnostic imaging of the intestine, especially regarding acute conditions.

The articles in this issue of *Radiologic Clinics of North America* on the Diagnostic Imaging of Intestinal Ischemia and Infarction are reviews written by authors personally and deeply involved in this area. The imaging findings of intestinal ischemia and disease progression to infarction are discussed for the small and large bowel, considering the arterial and venous etiology. There are also contributions on differential diagnosis and on conditions related to ischemia from bowel obstruction. In addition to imaging, reviews on etiology, pathogenesis, and clinical symptoms are included.

I am grateful to all of the outstanding contributors for their work and to Barton Dudlick for his assistance. It was a great privilege and honor to be Guest Editor for this issue of *Radiologic Clinics of North America*. I hope that you enjoy the content.

Stefania Romano, MD
Department of Diagnostic Imaging
Section of General and Emergency Radiology
A. Cardarelli Hospital
Naples, Italy

E-mail address:
stefromano@libero.it (S. Romano)

Radiol Clin N Am 46 (2008) xi
doi:10.1016/j.rcl.2008.08.003

Imaging in Intestinal Ischemic Disorders

Richard M. Gore, MD[a],*, Vahid Yaghmai, MD[b], Kiran H. Thakrar, MD[a],
Jonathan W. Berlin, MD[a], Uday K. Mehta, MD[a],
Geraldine M. Newmark, MD[a], Frank H. Miller, MD[b]

KEYWORDS

- Mesenteric ischemia • Mesenteric infarction
- Ischemic colitis • CT small bowel • CT colon

Gastrointestinal tract ischemia and infarction are a heterogeneous group of disorders (**Tables 1** and **2**) that have as their unifying theme hypoxia of the small bowel or colon. Ischemic bowel disease results from acute or chronic insufficiency of blood flow to the gut and includes acute and chronic small bowel and colonic ischemia (CI) in addition to infarction. Vascular compromise of the gut is a complex multifaceted condition that depends on the (1) state of the systemic circulation, (2) degree of functional or anatomic vascular compromise, (3) number and caliber of vessels affected, (4) response of the vascular bed to diminished perfusion, (5) nature and capacity of the collateral circulation, (6) duration of the ischemic insult, and (7) metabolic requirements of the involved segment of bowel.[1–12]

Patients who have intestinal ischemic disorders most often present with abdominal pain and other nonspecific symptoms, such as nausea, vomiting, diarrhea, and bloating. The diagnosis of mesenteric ischemia (MI) is often one of exclusion after more common possibilities, including bowel obstruction, appendicitis, diverticulitis, cholelithiasis, peptic ulcer disease, and gastroenteritis, have been excluded. Accordingly, a high index of clinical and radiologic suspicion is required to make a timely diagnosis of ischemia and infarction of the gut.[1–12]

Gastrointestinal tract ischemia can threaten bowel viability with potentially catastrophic consequences, including intestinal necrosis and gangrene. Dramatic improvements in cross-sectional imaging have the potential to afford earlier and more precise diagnosis, which is key to the reducing the morbidity and mortality of this potentially fatal condition.[1–12]

EPIDEMIOLOGY

Vascular compromise of the gut is responsible for approximately 0.1% of all hospital admissions and 1.0% of admissions for an acute abdomen. The diagnosis of this disorder is on the increase for several reasons. MI and infarction occur predominantly in the geriatric population with comorbid cardiovascular disease and other systemic dysfunction. The population is aging, and the number of cases of MI is expected to increase dramatically as the "Baby Boom" generation comes of age. Other factors include improved diagnostic techniques, heightened awareness of this diagnosis, and the efficacy of intensive care units to salvage critically ill patients.[13–28]

The causes of MI are protean (**Boxes 1–3**). Bowel ischemia most commonly occurs within the sixth and seventh decades of life. The age of onset depends on patient gender and the etiology of the ischemia. Primary mesenteric venous thrombosis (MVT) and nonocclusive mesenteric ischemia (NOMI) present at the ages of 66.5 and 63 years, respectively.[8] Superior mesenteric artery (SMA) occlusion and nonprimary MVT present nearly a decade later, at the ages of 77.5 and

[a] Department of Radiology, Evanston Northwestern Healthcare, Northwestern University Medical School, 2650 Ridge Avenue, Evanston, IL 60201, USA
[b] Department of Radiology, Northwestern Memorial Hospital, Northwestern University Medical School, 676 St. Clair Street, Chicago, IL 60611, USA
* Corresponding author.
E-mail address: rmgore1953@aol.com (R.M. Gore).

Radiol Clin N Am 46 (2008) 845–875
doi:10.1016/j.rcl.2008.05.004
0033-8389/08/$ – see front matter © 2008 Elsevier Inc. All rights reserved.

Table 1
Types and approximate incidences of intestinal ischemia

Colonic ischemia	75%
Acute mesenteric ischemia	25%
Focal mesenteric ischemia	5%
Chronic mesenteric ischemia	5%
Mesenteric venous thrombosis	Included in previous incidences

74 years, respectively.[8] Chronic mesenteric ischemia (CMI) presents in younger patients than those with acute mesenteric ischemia (AMI), with a female prevalence as high as 4:1. This is in contrast to the overwhelming prevalence of men with peripheral vascular and aneurysmal disease. Generally, women present with ischemia at an earlier age than their male counterparts, which may contribute to the overall earlier age of onset of CMI.[13–28]

Prompt diagnosis of MI is facilitated by recognizing the various risk factors and comorbidities. Although there is significant overlap among the risk factors for the various vascular disorders of the intestines, certain etiology-specific risk factors have been described.

AMI has been linked to congestive heart failure, valvular heart disease, cardiac arrhythmias, low cardiac output states, recent myocardial infarction, intra-abdominal malignancies, and emboli to the extremities.[22] There is a greater than 50% association between CMI and coronary artery disease, peripheral vascular disease, hypertension, and smoking. Tobacco use is strongly associated with gut ischemia, with some 70% to 90% of patients admitting to significant use. Other comorbidities include diabetes, hypertension, renal disease, malignancy, gastrointestinal disease, and hypercoagulable states.[6–9]

INTESTINAL VASCULAR ANATOMY

Knowledge of mesenteric vascular anatomy and physiology is key to an appreciation of the causes and consequences of intestinal ischemia and infarction. The anatomy of the mesenteric circulation is complicated by the almost endless variations of blood supply to the gut.

Celiac Axis

The celiac artery (**Fig. 1**) is the largest branch of the abdominal aorta, and it supplies the embryologic foregut. It leaves the abdominal aorta at an angle of 90° at the level of the T12 or L1 vertebral body. After coursing ventrally and inferiorly 1 to 2 cm, the celiac artery branches into the common hepatic, splenic, and left gastric arteries in 75% of the population. In 25%, there is a true trifurcation of these vessels, and in 1%, there is a common origin of the celiac and superior mesenteric branches—the celiacomesenteric trunk.[16]

The common hepatic artery gives rise to the gastroduodenal artery, which then becomes the right gastroepiploic artery and the anterior and posterior superior pancreaticoduodenal arteries. Typically, the splenic artery gives off the left gastroepiploic artery, which joins the right gastroepiploic artery. The left gastric artery anastomoses with the right gastric artery along the lesser curvature of the stomach.[16]

Superior Mesenteric Artery

The SMA (**Fig. 2**) is a large-caliber structure with a narrow takeoff from the aorta, making it the most susceptible of the major mesenteric vessels to embolic phenomena. It supplies the entire embryologic midgut and is the second largest intra-abdominal branch of the aorta. As a general rule, there are more SMA branches to the distal small bowel than the more proximal portions,

Table 2
Causes and approximate incidences of acute mesenteric ischemia

Superior mesenteric artery embolus	50%
Nonocclusive mesenteric ischemia	25%
Superior mesenteric artery thrombosis	10%
Mesenteric venous thrombosis	10%
Focal segmental ischemia	5%

The middle colic artery typically arises from the proximal SMA to supply the transverse colon and communicates with branches of the inferior mesenteric artery (IMA). The splenic flexure of the colon is a watershed region between these two mesenteric circulations. Accordingly, it is a frequent sight of ischemic colitis.

The right colic artery, which supplies the middle to distal ascending colon, usually arises from a common trunk with or just inferior to the middle colic artery.

Box 1
Causes of mesenteric ischemia

AMI

Emboli

   Arrhythmias

   Valvular disease

   Myocardial infarction

   Hypokinetic ventricular wall

   Cardiac aneurysm

   Aortic atherosclerotic disease

   Iatrogenic

Thrombosis

   Atherosclerotic disease

Nonocclusive

   Heart failure

   Cardiac bypass

   Sepsis

   Renal failure

   Medications

   Pancreatitis

   Burns

Venous occlusion

   Hypercoagulable states

   Sepsis

   Malignancy

   Portal hypertension

   Compression

   Pregnancy

CMI

   Atherosclerotic disease

   Arterial hyperplasia or dysplasia

   Inflammatory disease

Box 2
Disorders associated with mesenteric venous thrombosis

Hypercoagulable states

   Activated protein C resistance

   Antithrombin resistance

   Protein C deficiency

   Protein S deficiency

   Methyltetrahydrofolate deficiency

   Estrogen use (oral contraceptive, hormone replacement therapy)

   Polycythemia vera

   Thrombocytosis

   Neoplasms

Peripheral deep vein thrombosis

Pregnancy

Portal hypertension

   Cirrhosis

   Congestive splenomegaly

   After sclerotherapy of esophageal varices

Inflammation

   Diverticulitis

   Appendicitis

   Pancreatitis

   Perforated viscus

   Inflammatory bowel disease

   Pelvic or intra-abdominal abscess

Postoperative state or trauma

   Blunt abdominal trauma

   Splenectomy and other postoperative states

Decompression sickness

---

providing greater potential for distal anastomoses.[12,26]

The SMA originates 1 cm beneath the level of the celiac artery, usually at the level of L1, and courses inferiorly toward the right and terminates as the ileocolic artery at the level of the cecum. The major branches of the SMA are the inferior pancreaticoduodenal artery, the middle colic artery, the right colic artery, 4 to 6 jejunal branches, and 9 to 13 ileal branches.[16]

Box 3
Causes of colonic ischemia

Inferior mesenteric artery thrombosis

Arterial embolism

Cholesterol emboli

Cardiac arrhythmia

Congestive heart failure

Shock

Volvulus

Strangulated hernia

Vasculitis

Hematologic disorders

  Sickle cell anemia

  Protein C and S deficiencies

  Antithrombin III deficiency

  Factor V Leiden mutation (activated protein C resistance)

  Factor I 2010A mutation (in combination with oral contraceptive use)

  Polycythemia vera

Infections

  Parasites

    Angiostrongylus costaricensis

    Entamoeba histolytica

  Viruses

    Cytomegalovirus

  Bacteria

    Escherichia coli O157:H7

Trauma

Long-distance running

Pregnancy

Surgical

  Aneurysmectomy

  Aortoiliac reconstruction

  Gynecologic operations

  Exchange transfusion

  Colonic bypass

  Lumbar aortography

  Colectomy with IMA ligation

  Colonoscopy

Medications

  Related to vasoconstriction or vasculitis

    Digitalis

    Vasopressin

    Gold

    Pseudoephedrine

    Sumatriptan

    Cocaine

    Methamphetamine

    Nonsteroidal anti-inflammatory drugs

    Imipramine

  Related to hypovolemia or constipation

    Interferon-α

    Saline laxatives

    Estrogens

    Progestins

    Danazol

    Psychotropic medications

    Alosetron

Inferior Mesenteric Artery

The IMA (**Fig. 3**) is the smallest of the mesenteric vessels and arises 6 to 7 cm below the SMA at the level of L3. It supplies the hindgut: the distal transverse colon, splenic flexure, descending colon, and rectosigmoid. The IMA is a narrow-caliber artery (0.5 cm) that has a relatively acute takeoff angle from the aorta, rendering it much less susceptible to embolic events. The major branches of the IMA include the left colic, sigmoid, and hemorrhoidal arteries. The ascending branches of the left colic artery reach the splenic flexure in 80% to 85% of patients and extend to the midtransverse colon in 15% to 20% of individuals. At this point, they anastomose with branches of the middle colic artery from the SMA. The sigmoidal branches form arcades that anastomose with the left colic artery and superior hemorrhoidal artery. The superior hemorrhoidal artery supplies blood to the wall of the upper two thirds of the rectum and to the mucosa of the lower third of the rectum.[12,16]

The middle hemorrhoidal artery arises from the anterior division of the internal iliac artery or from the vesical branch of this vessel. The middle hemorrhoidal artery traverses the infraperitoneal pelvis in the lateral ligaments and supplies the middle third of the rectum. The inferior hemorrhoidal artery is also a branch of the anterior division of the internal iliac artery. It is invested by endopelvic fascia as it exits the pelvis, below the piriformis muscle, through the greater sciatic foramen. It pursues a short course in the buttock and then

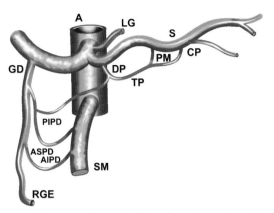

Fig. 1. Diagram of typical celiac axis anatomy. A, aorta; AIPD, anterior inferior pancreaticoduodenal artery; ASPD, anterior superior pancreaticoduodenal artery; C, celiac axis; CP, caudal pancreatic artery; DP, dorsal pancreatic artery; GD, gastroduodenal artery; H, common hepatic artery; LG, left gastric artery; PIPD, posterior inferior pancreaticoduodenal artery; PM, pancreata magna; RGE, right gastroepiploic artery; S, splenic artery; SM, superior mesenteric artery; TP, transverse pancreatic artery. (*From* Nebesar RA, Kornblith PL, Pollard JJ, et al. Celiac and superior mesenteric arteries: a correlation of angiograms and dissections. Boston: Little, Brown; 1969. p. 45; with permission.)

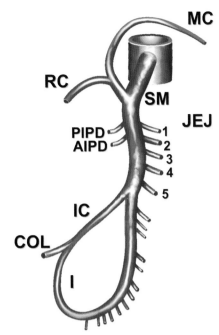

Fig. 2. Diagram of typical superior mesenteric artery anatomy. A, aorta; AIPD, anterior inferior pancreaticoduodenal artery; COL, colic branches; I, ileal branches; IC, ileocolic artery; JEJ, jejunal branches; MC, middle colic artery; PIPD, posterior inferior pancreaticoduodenal artery; RC, right colic artery; SM, superior mesenteric artery. (*From* Nebesar RA, Kornblith PL, Pollard JJ, et al. Celiac and superior mesenteric arteries: a correlation of angiograms and dissections. Boston: Little, Brown; 1969. p. 48; with permission.)

re-enters the pelvis. It crosses the ischiorectal fossa, which may cause considerable bleeding if encountered during abdominoperineal resection of the rectum. This vessel supplies the levator ani and sphincters in addition to the lower rectum and anal canal.[12–16] The mesenteric vascular anatomy is well depicted on cross-sectional imaging (**Fig. 4**).

Mesenteric Collateral Flow Patterns

There are numerous sources of collateral flow between the mesenteric vessels and nonmesenteric systemic vessels. This redundancy imparts substantial protection against intestinal ischemia and infarction after segmental vascular occlusion. As a result of these multiple potential sources of collateral flow, at least two of the three main vessels must be occluded or have critical stenoses for MI to develop.

Celiac axis–superior mesenteric artery collaterals

At autopsy, approximately 20% of individuals have greater than 50% stenosis of the celiac artery.[14,15] Most of these patients are asymptomatic because of the rich collateral vessels from the SMA (**Fig. 5**). The gastroduodenal and superior and inferior pancreaticoduodenal arteries are the primary potential pathways of collateral flow between the celiac axis

and SMA. The arc of Barkow forms potential communications between omental branches from the SMA and branches of the celiac axis.

Superior mesenteric artery–inferior mesenteric artery collaterals

At autopsy, it is not uncommon for the SMA (30%) and IMA (30%) to be stenotic[14,15] The marginal artery of Drummond, which lies in the subperitoneal space of the mesocolon of the descending colon, consists of branches from the ileocolic, right, middle, and left colic arteries. An anastomosis between the middle and left colic arteries is present in 95% of individuals and occurs at the splenic flexure—the so-called "Griffith's point." The arc of Riolan (meandering mesenteric artery) lies within the descending mesocolon as well but is more centrally located and usually joins the middle and left colic arteries.[12,16]

Inferior mesenteric artery–systemic circulation collaterals

There are collateral vessels within the rectum by way of the anastomoses of the superior rectal

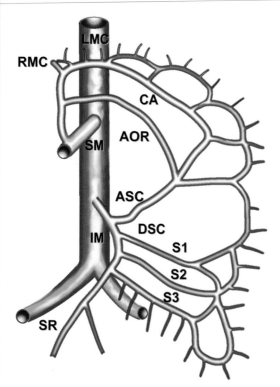

Fig. 3. Diagram of typical IMA anatomy. AOR, arc of Riolan; ASC, ascending branch of the left colic artery; CA, central artery; DSC, descending branch of the left colic artery; IM, inferior mesenteric artery; LMC, left branch of middle colic artery; MA, marginal artery of Drummond; MC, middle colic artery; RMC, right branch of middle colic artery; S1, S2, and S3, sigmoid branches; SM, superior mesenteric artery; SR, superior rectal artery. (*From* Nebesar RA, Kornblith PL, Pollard JJ, et al. Celiac and superior mesenteric arteries: a correlation of angiograms and dissections. Boston: Little, Brown; 1969. p. 49; with permission.)

(hemorrhoidal) arteries with the middle and inferior rectal arteries, which originate from the internal iliac blood vessels. The three hemorrhoidal vessels form a comprehensive anastomotic network in the submucosa of the anal canal and lower rectum. This complex blood supply to the rectum with its redundancies and collaterals explains why the rectum is often spared in patients who have bowel ischemia and infarction.

Clinical correlates of mesenteric anatomy

Chronic blockage of any single mesenteric artery is usually inconsequential if the collateral pathways are functional. Critical ischemia from acute occlusion can result from single-vessel disease in the absence of adequate collaterals or when multiple vessels are diseased.[12–16]

Certain operative procedures can disrupt key mesenteric collaterals. In a patient who has chronic celiac artery occlusion, a Whipple's operation can cause hepatic ischemia by interrupting collateral arterial flow from the SMA through the pancreaticoduodenal arcades. A segmental colectomy may interrupt critical anastomotic networks between the SMA and IMA and result in acute ischemia in patients who have severe mesenteric occlusive disease.

The IMA is the most frequently occluded mesenteric vessel by chronic vascular disease. This artery is usually sacrificed during abdominal aortic aneurysm repair. If the SMA is severely diseased and the midgut is receiving a large proportion of blood from the arc of Riolan, sacrificing this vessel during aneurysm repair can cause small bowel and right colon infarction.[16]

PHYSIOLOGY OF THE MESENTERIC CIRCULATION

In the fasting state, the mesenteric vessels receive approximately 20% to 25% of the cardiac output and the splanchnic circulation contains approximately one third of the total blood volume, which makes it the circulatory system's largest reservoir. Approximately 25% of the splanchnic circulation flows directly to the liver by way of the hepatic artery, and the remaining 75% of blood flow reaches the liver by way of the portal venous system.[12,16]

At rest, approximately 70% to 80% of the blood flow is directed to the mucosa, 15% to 25% is distributed to the muscularis propria and serosal layers, and 5% is distributed to the submucosal layer. The epithelial cells in the terminal villi receive 60% of the mucosal blood flow, with the crypts and goblet cells receiving the other 40%.[14,15]

CLASSIFICATION OF ISCHEMIC BOWEL DISEASE

Intestinal ischemic disorders have been classified into several major types:[17–19]

    AMI
        SMAE
        NOMI
        Superior mesenteric artery thrombosis
        Superior mesenteric vein thrombosis
    CMI (intestinal angina)
    CI
        Reversible ischemic colopathy
        Transient ulcerating ischemic colitis
        Chronic ulcerating ischemic colitis
        Colonic stricture
        Colonic gangrene
        Fulminant universal ischemic colitis

CI is the most common vascular disorder of the gut, followed by AMI. AMI is associated with compromise of the blood flow in the SMA distribution

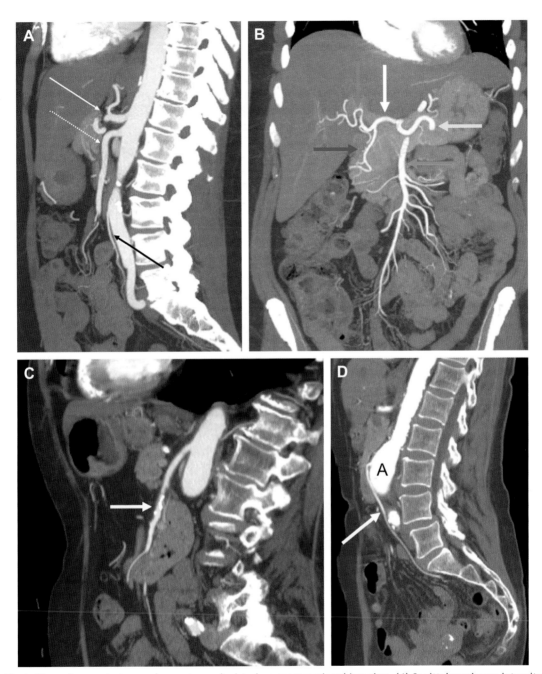

Fig. 4. Normal mesenteric vascular anatomy depicted on cross-sectional imaging. (*A*) Sagittal maximum intensity projection (MIP) multidetector CT (MDCT) image demonstrates the origins of the celiac artery (*solid white arrow*), superior mesenteric artery (SMA) (*broken white arrow*), and IMA (*black arrow*). (*B*) Coronal reformatted MIP MDCT image nicely depicts the jejunal branches of the SMA (*red arrow*). The splenic artery (*yellow arrow*), common hepatic artery (*white arrow*), gastroduodenal artery (*blue arrow*), and proper hepatic artery (*green arrow*) are also shown. (*C*) Sagittal reformatted MDCT image shows atherosclerotic calcification (*white arrow*) in the SMA. (*D*) Sagittal reformatted MDCT image shows the IMA (*white arrow*) originating from an abdominal aortic aneurysm (*A*). (*E*) Coronal reformatted MDCT image demonstrates the superior mesenteric vein (SMV) (*white arrow*) and its major tributaries. (*F*) Gray-scale sagittal sonogram of the abdominal aorta reveals the origins of the celiac artery (*broken arrow*) and SMA (*solid arrow*). (*G*) MR imaging venogram shows the mesenteric circulation in a patient who has cirrhosis and portal hypertension. The white arrow indicates the portal vein, the yellow arrow indicates the SMV, and the red arrow indicates the splenic vein. (*Courtesy of* Dr. Jochen A. Gaa, Munich, Germany.)

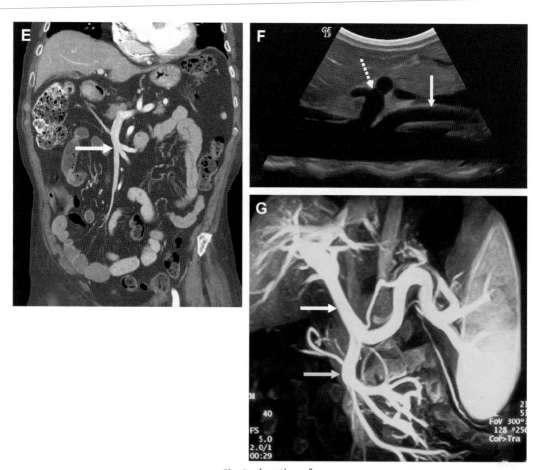

Fig. 4. (*continued*)

affecting all or portions of the small bowel and right colon. In CMI, the splanchnic circulation is insufficient in meeting the functional demands of the gut but there is no loss of tissue viability. AMI, CMI, and CI have distinct clinical manifestations that require different management strategies. The differentiation among these various ischemic disorders can be made in some patients with the assistance of cross-sectional imaging.

PATHOLOGIC FINDINGS OF INTESTINAL ISCHEMIA
Small Bowel

Pathologic evidence of small bowel ischemia and infarction (**Figs. 6–8**) may be diffuse and confluent or patchy and multifocal. The serosal aspect of the affected small bowel often appears congested or blue and black. Perforations may be present but may not be accompanied by well-developed fibrinous exudates if the surgical resection occurs within a short time of presentation. The mesentery is usually pale in arterial occlusions and congested and hemorrhagic in venous thrombosis. The demarcation between normal and involved gut is usually abrupt. The intestinal lumen is invariably filled with blood, and the mucosal surface may appear beefy red, boggy, and ulcerated and may contain irregularly protruding mucosal islands. This mucosal appearance is responsible for the "thumbprinting" sign. Pseudomembranes and transmural hemorrhage may be seen. The wall of the involved segment is often friable and thin. In patients who have mesenteric vein thrombosis, thrombi can be seen in mesenteric veins on gross examination.[14,15]

Early histologic changes consist of hemorrhage, congestion, and edema of the submucosa, sometimes associated with preservation of the overlying mucosa. Submucosal changes can then lead to various degrees of mucosal necrosis with or without ulceration, luminal hemorrhage, and pseudomembrane formation. In the acute setting, there is absence of a chronic inflammatory response, although neutrophils may be seen if enough time has elapsed since the onset of occlusion.[14,15]

The mucosa shows a loss of epithelium, which occurs progressively from the tips of the villi to the base of the crypts and is associated with

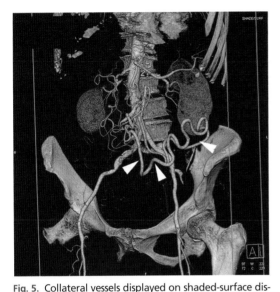

Fig. 5. Collateral vessels displayed on shaded-surface display multidectector CT (MDCT) image. The marginal artery of Drummond (*arrowheads*) in a patient who has SMA stenosis demonstrates the collateral pathways between the IMA and SMA. (*From* Horton KM, Fishman EK. Vascular disorders of the small bowel. In: Gore RM, Levine MS, editors. Textbook of gastrointestinal radiology. 3rd edition. Philadelphia: WB Saunders; 2008. p. 909.)

various degrees of edema and congestion. Within hours of the injury, neutrophils influx into the damaged area. Depending on the extent and severity of the injury, the mucosal changes may reverse to normal if the ischemic insult stops. If the ischemia is persistent or severe, tissue healing may result in fibrosis and stricture formation.[14,15]

Mesenteric vessel evaluation may be confusing, because thrombi may form acutely as a response to stasis and congestion. Clinically significant thrombi show evidence of organization, implying their presence over a significant period. Fibrin thrombi may be present in small arterioles in areas of necrosis and do not, by themselves, indicate vasculitis or a hypercoagulable state.[14,15]

Colon

Acute ischemic lesions of the colon show necrosis of the superficial portion of the mucosa that often spares the deeper portions of the colonic crypts. The remaining crypts typically have an atrophic or withered appearance that reveals striking cytologic atypia, which may be mistaken for dysplasia. Pseudomembranes, hemorrhage into the lamina propria, and hyalinization of the lamina propria may also be seen. These lesions may regress on

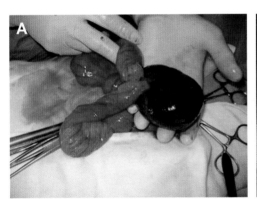

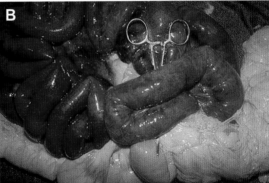

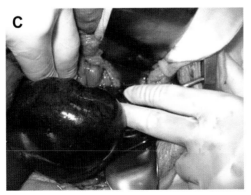

Fig. 6. Pathologic findings of intestinal ischemia and infarction: intraoperative images. (*A*) Short segment of small bowel infarction attributable to strangulation from closed-loop obstruction caused by an adhesive band. (*B*) Long segment of small bowel infarction caused by SMA occlusion. (*C*) Sigmoid colon infarction attributable to a volvulus.

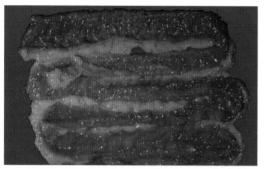

Fig. 7. Pathologic findings of intestinal ischemia and infarction: gross pathologic image. The mucosa demonstrates marked hyperemia and hemorrhage.

their own, or frank gangrene with perforation or stricture formation may occur.[14,15]

The chronic phase of CI may be more difficult to diagnose, because the only histologic findings may be areas of submucosal fibrosis and stricture, which are nonspecific.[14,15]

CLINICAL FEATURES OF MESENTERIC ISCHEMIA

To date, no reliable physiologic or biochemical means of detecting MI and predicting behavior have been established. Serum lactate is an established marker of cell hypoxia but lactic acidosis is often a late finding in the diagnostic pathway with

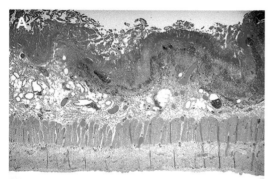

Fig. 8. Pathologic findings of intestinal ischemia and infarction: histopathology of ischemic enteritis. (*A*) Mucosal surface of the bowel shows early necrosis with hyperemia extending from the mucosa to submucosal and muscular wall vessels. The submucosa and muscularis mucosa, however, are still intact. (*B*) At higher magnification with more advanced necrosis, the small intestinal mucosa shows hemorrhage with acute inflammation.

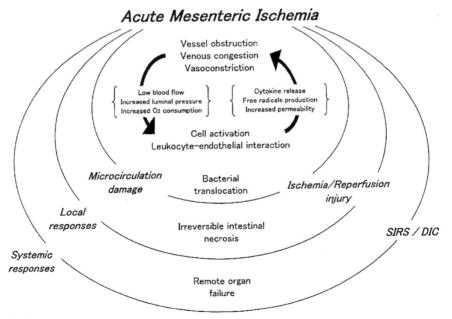

Fig. 9. Local and systemic responses in AMI. DIC, disseminated intravascular coagulation; SIRS, systemic inflammatory response syndrome. (*From* Yasuhara H. Acute mesenteric ischemia: the challenge of gastroenterology. Surg Today 2005;35:187; with permission.)

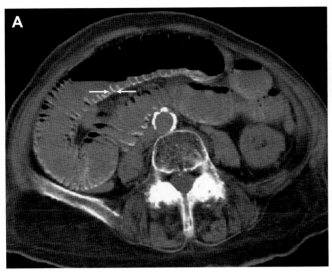
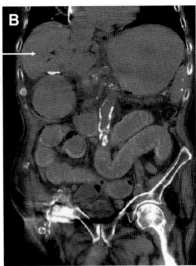

Fig. 10. Intramural hemorrhage associated with acute superior mesenteric arterial compromise. Axial (*A*) and coronal reformatted (*B*) MDCT images obtained without oral or intravenous contrast material demonstrate dilated fluid-filled small bowel. The wall (*arrows*) in A is hyperdense and thin, indicating intramural hemorrhage. No reperfusion has occurred. There is intrahepatic portal venous gas (*arrow*) in B.

concomitant shock, bowel necrosis, and circulatory collapse.[22,26]

Recently, plasma D-dimer levels have been suggested as an early marker of acute ischemia. In animal studies, they have been shown to correlate with the onset of ischemia and function as a time-sensitive indicator of disease progression.[20] The enzyme alcohol dehydrogenase has been identified as a time-sensitive indicator of bowel ischemia as opposed to generalized systemic hypoperfusion. Glutathione S-transferase is released with cell membrane damage, and several isoforms have been correlated with bowel specificity. This detoxifying cytosolic enzyme has been shown to exhibit a time- and duration-specific detectable increase with progressive tissue ischemia.[4,20]

Acute Mesenteric Ischemia

The diagnosis of AMI can be difficult, because most patients have nonspecific symptoms of abdominal pain. Abdominal pain out of proportion to the findings on physical examination and

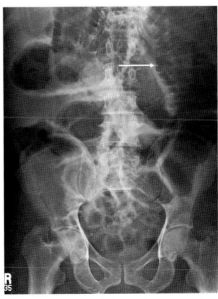

Fig. 11. Intramural hemorrhage associated with acute mesenteric venous compromise. MDCT shows mural thickening of the small bowel with submucosal edema and a hyperdense mucosa, producing a target appearance (*arrows*). Note the ascites (A) and increased intraluminal fluid.

Fig. 12. Reflex ileus. Abdominal plain radiograph shows dilated segments of the jejunum in a patient who has MI. Note the thickened valvulae conniventes (*arrow*).

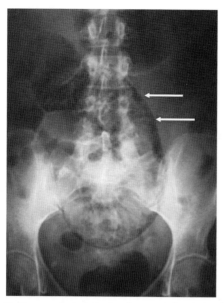

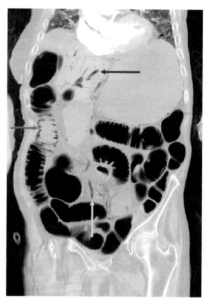

Fig. 13. Pneumatosis intestinalis on plain abdominal radiograph. Multiple linear intramural lucencies (*arrows*) are present within the small bowel in this patient who has strangulated small bowel obstruction attributable to a ventral hernia. Necrotic bowel was resected at the time of surgery.

Fig. 15. Pneumatosis intestinalis attributable to small bowel infarction in an elderly patient who has cardiac arrhythmias. Coronal reformatted MDCT image shows intramural gas (*red arrow*) in several ileal segments. Mesenteric (*yellow arrow*) and intrahepatic (*blue arrow*) portal venous gas is also evident.

persisting beyond 2 to 3 hours is the classic presentation. Nausea, diarrhea, vomiting, and anorexia can also be part of the initial symptom complex. An elevated white blood cell count is common; 15% of patients report melena or

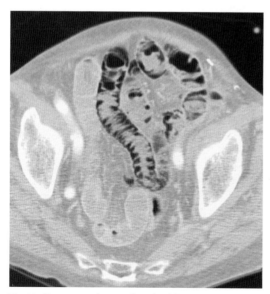

Fig. 14. Pneumatosis associated with mesenteric arterial compromise. MDCT scan of the pelvis displayed at lung windows demonstrates pneumatosis involving several ileal loops.

hematochezia, and occult fecal blood is found in 50%. With delay in diagnosis and progression to full-thickness mural injury, the patient develops peritoneal signs of distention, guarding, rigidity, and hypotension. Lactic acidosis is present in addition to elevations in serum amylase, aspartate aminotransferase, and creatine phosphokinase. If hyperkalemia and hyperphosphatemia are present, bowel infarction should be suspected.[1,3,6,26]

An oxygen supply that is insufficient to meet the demands of the gut results in increased production of lactate by the bowel as a result of anaerobic glycolysis within cells. MI also increases xanthinoxidase within small bowel mucosa, which converts hypoxanthine to uric acid. The free radicals that form with reperfusion damage the cytomembrane, and cell edema ensues with cellular decay (**Fig. 9**).

There are four clinical-radiologic stages that occur in patients who have ischemia and infarction of the gut.[4,20,25,27,28]

First stage
Immediately after arterial occlusion, there is rapid onset of severe abdominal pain associated with loose and sometimes bloody stools and vomiting. Typically, there is discordance in the severe, often excruciating, degree of abdominal pain and a relative paucity of physical abdominal findings. At this point, hyperperistalsis and hyperactive bowel sounds on auscultation are evident. The plain abdominal radiograph may show a gasless

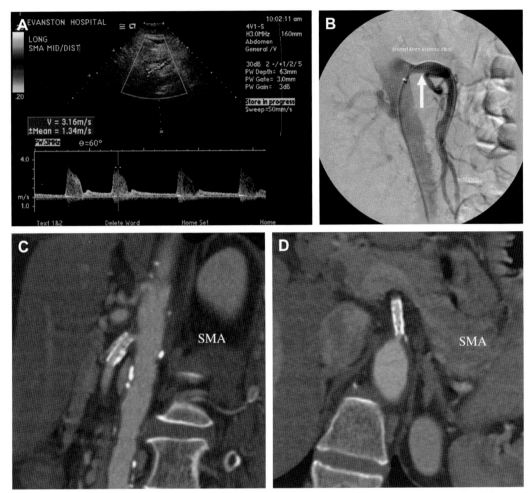

Fig. 16. SMA stenosis in a patient who has chronic intestinal angina treated with a vascular stent. (A) Doppler ultrasound analysis shows a markedly elevated SMA peak systolic velocity of 3.16 m/s. The waveform also shows spectral broadening. (B) Lateral angiographic image shows deployment of the stent (arrow) through the stenotic portion of the SMA. Curved reformatted axial (C) and sagittal reformatted (D) MDCT images show the stent at the origin of the SMA. Note the atherosclerotic calcification of the aorta.

abdomen. Thrombus may be seen in cases of superior mesenteric artery thrombosis (SMAT) and superior mesenteric artery embolism (SMAE) but may be relatively normal in cases of NOMI.[27,28]

In patients who have acute MVT, plain abdominal radiographs may reveal a reflex ileus pattern without bowel distention. Sonography may show a homogeneously hypoechoic intestinal wall as a result of edema that occurs earlier in the course of disease when compared with SMA compromise.[27,28]

Second stage

In this stage, the pain may be diminishing but becomes more continuous and diffuse. The abdomen becomes distended, and there is more generalized tenderness. Bowel sounds are absent. With persistent arterial occlusion, there is disruption of the microvascular integrity of the bowel wall. The capillary walls become damaged because they derive oxygen by direct diffusion from the blood pool. This increases mucosal permeability so that the remaining blood may extravasate, causing hemorrhagic foci in the thinned bowel wall (Fig. 10). Pari passu, the mucosa cannot produce the normal amount and quality of enteric secretions and the intestinal microflora can proliferate, producing gas.[27,28]

Plain abdominal radiographs may show mild gaseous dilation of the affected loops, which have lost their tone. Multidetector CT (MDCT) demonstrates these findings in addition to a "paper-thin" bowel wall with decreased mural enhancement. If reperfusion does not occur, transmural bowel necrosis may ensue and intramural air may dissect into the necrotic mucosa; from there, it may dissect intramurally, subperitoneally, and into the

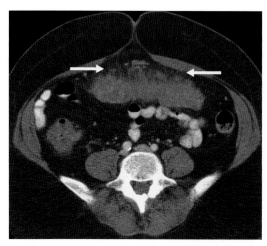

Fig. 17. Colonic ischemia in a 26-year-old woman who has polyarteritis nodosa. MDCT reveals mural thickening of the transverse and, to a lesser degree, ascending colon with submucosal edema. Note the pericolic streaky densities (*arrows*).

peritoneal cavity and ultimately spread through the mesenteric and portal venous system.[27,28]

With persistent mesenteric venous occlusion, the intramural blood volume increases as arterial blood keeps flowing into the bowel wall in patients with venous compromise. This leads to increased intravascular hydrostatic pressure, which dilates the blood vessels and widens the fenestrations among the vascular endothelial cells. This leads to extravasation of plasma, contrast material, or red blood cells (**Fig. 11**) into the bowel wall or lumen. Tension in the submucosal extravascular compartment or prolonged stasis-induced thrombosis of the microvasculature may interrupt arterial blood flow. The imaging findings at this stage of disease are related to mural thickening, intramural hemorrhage, and submucosal edema.[27,28]

Sonography may reveal thrombus at the origin of the superior mesenteric vein (SMV) and mural thickening with hyperechoic mucosal layers and hypoechoic submucosa attributable to edema of the affected loops.

On MDCT, the ischemic gut demonstrates a target appearance with an inner hyperdense ring as a result of surface mucosal hypervascularity, hemorrhage, and ulceration; a middle hypodense edematous submucosa; and a normal or slightly thickened muscularis propria. The damage to the gut may be reversible at this stage of impaired venous drainage, because the integrity of the deeper mural layers is preserved. If the vascular compromise persists, three possible outcomes may ensue: healing, chronic ischemia, or progression to intestinal infarction. Healing may lead to

stricture formation because of circumferential granulation tissue formation and fibrosis in response to parietal layer damage.

Third stage

With progressive mural injury, fluid, protein, and electrolytes begin to leak into the lumen, the bowel becomes necrotic, and peritonitis develops. Fluid loss can be massive, and this stage of ischemia is clinically similar in its manifestations to other causes of generalized peritonitis.

If the arterial blood flow compromise is alleviated, reperfusion of the gut is associated with several radiographic findings best seen with MDCT. Blood, plasma, contrast material, or red blood cells may extravasate through the disrupted vascular wall into the mucosa and submucosa, causing mural thickening and bloody fluid filling the intestinal lumen. Plain abdominal radiographs may show mild dilation of the affected loops, with mural thickening, sparse and subtle valvulae conniventes, and some air-fluid levels. Ultrasound examination may reveal increased intraluminal secretions and decreased peristalsis.[27,28]

On MDCT, the thickened submucosa may be hyperdense because of hemorrhage. After contrast administration, the mucosa may show hyperenhancement with submucosal edema and hypodensity. Mural stratification typically is preserved.

Persistent venous thrombosis leads to mesenteric vascular engorgement and edema, with the formation of venous collateral blood vessels. This stage produces imaging findings typical of patients with chronic venous impairment. CT shows mural thickening of the involved segments, peritoneal fluid, and mesenteric engorgement.

Fourth stage

Abdominal plain radiographs show markedly dilated loops with thickening of the valvulae conniventes and multiple air-fluid levels (**Fig. 12**). Extraluminal fluid and absent peristalsis are evident sonographically. CT may demonstrate SMA thrombosis or emboli; bowel enhancement is poor, and pneumatosis may be evident in cases of frank mural necrosis.[27,28]

Frank intestinal infarction initially causes progressive submucosal hemorrhage and edema. The cyanosis leads to loss of integrity of the intestinal wall with necrosis and peritonitis. Intramural and mesenteric venous gas may be apparent, associated with subperitoneal or intraperitoneal serosanguineous or bloody fluid.

Conventional abdominal radiographs may show mural thickening, pneumatosis (**Fig. 13**), or pneumoperitoneum. Sonography reveals mural

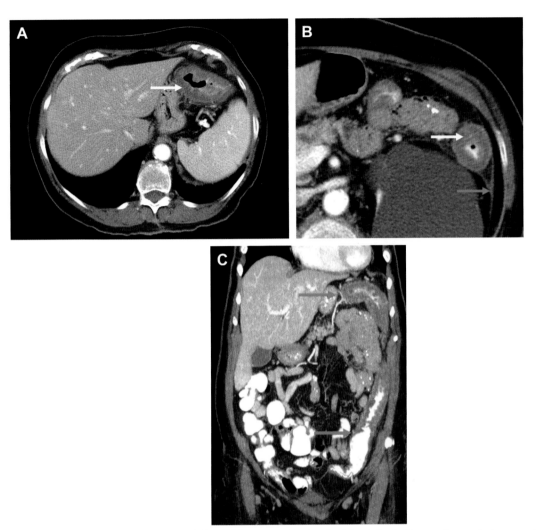

Fig. 18. Ischemic colitis: MDCT findings. (*A*) Axial image at the level of the splenic flexure demonstrates mural thickening and submucosal edema (*white arrow*). (*B*) More caudal scan shows that the proximal descending colon has a target appearance with higher density mucosa and muscularis mucosa framing the edematous submucosa (*white arrow*). A small amount of fluid is seen in the fascial trifurcation (*red arrow*) of the left subperitoneal space. (*C*) Coronal reformatted image reveals the full extent (*red arrows*) of colonic involvement.

thickening of the involved segment, intramural or intraperitoneal gas, and peritoneal fluid. On CT, venous thrombosis, absence of mural enhancement, and the presence of fluid and gas may be evident in the mesenteric and portal veins, bowel wall, and subperitoneal or peritoneal space (**Figs. 14** and **15**).

Chronic Mesenteric Ischemia

This disorder, also known as abdominal angina (AA), is often insidious in its presentation (**Fig. 16**). The occlusive lesion compromises the increased blood flow that typically occurs after eating. This leads to postprandial pain that is maximal 30 to 90 minutes after food intake. The intensity of the pain leads to fear of food and weight loss, which is compensated for to some extent by frequent intake of small meals—the small meal syndrome. The appetite is usually not affected, which is an important distinguishing feature from patients who have cancer. Constipation is often present initially, but with the development of ischemic villous atrophy, malabsorption and diarrhea may develop.[5]

Colonic Ischemia and Infarction

Patients who have acute CI typically present with acute mild abdominal pain and tenderness over the affected bowel, most often on the left. Within 24 hours of the onset of abdominal pain, mild to

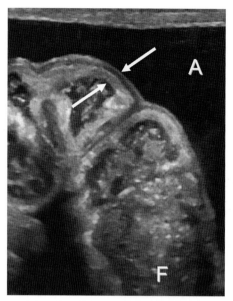

Fig. 19. Ischemic colitis: sonographic features. Mural thickening (*arrows*) of the colon is present associated with a large amount of ascites (A). Note the fecal material (F) and fluid within the colonic lumen.

moderate amounts of rectal bleeding or bloody diarrhea occur. Approximately one half of patients who have nongangrenous CI have complete resolution within 2 weeks, with recurrence developing in only 5% of individuals. Patients who have gangrenous colon ischemia and require surgical resection have greater than 50% mortality.[5,11,13]

There are three clinical-radiologic stages that occur in patients who have ischemia and infarction of the gut.[27,28]

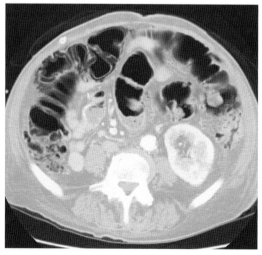

Fig. 20. Colon infarction on an MDCT scan displayed with lung windows. Pneumatosis is present within the right colon.

First stage

With early colonic arterial compromise, there is mural thickening and extensive submucosal edema. The colon has a shaggy contour (**Fig. 17**), and there is a variable degree of pericolonic streakiness and peritoneal fluid. In this phase, there is mucosal hyperdensity as a result of hemorrhage. This is more commonly seen in the left colon.

In the early stages of colonic venous compromise, there is mural thickening and mucosal hyperdensity from hemorrhagic phenomena. Moderate peritoneal fluid may be present, and occlusion of mesenteric vessels is visible.[27,28]

Second stage

In this phase of colonic arterial compromise, there is progression of the ischemic change without reperfusion. This causes symmetric and concentric mural thickening of the colon.

This phase of colonic venous compromise is associated with submucosal hypodensity attributable to mural edema (**Fig. 18**). The involved colon has a shaggy contour associated with pericolic streakiness, indicating progression of the impaired venous drainage. Peritoneal fluid (**Fig. 19**) of varying amounts accompanies this stage of CI. Mesenteric vascular occlusion can be visualized.[27,28]

Third stage

In this phase of arterial occlusion or hypoperfusion, there is frank infarction with intramural gas and mesenteric or portal venous gas. There is absence of a small amount of intraperitoneal fluid, absence of parietal enhancement, and pneumoperitoneum.[27,28]

With progressive vascular compromise, the colon becomes homogeneously thickened with decreased enhancement. Pneumatosis (**Fig. 20**) and portal (**Fig. 21**) and mesenteric venous gas may be present, and occlusion of mesenteric vessels can be identified.

Differential Diagnosis

The recognition of bowel ischemia and infarction can be difficult, because most patients present with nonspecific symptoms and signs. This is particularly true in patients who have other pressing clinical issues. Appendicitis, diverticulitis, nonstrangulating bowel obstruction, peptic ulcer disease, gastritis, gastroenteritis, infectious ileocolitis, inflammatory bowel disease, pancreatitis, acute cholecystis, and ruptured aortic aneurysm often enter the clinician's mind as the most likely diagnosis, with intestinal ischemia not considered or placed at the bottom of the differential diagnosis. Clearly, the diagnosis hinges on having a high index of

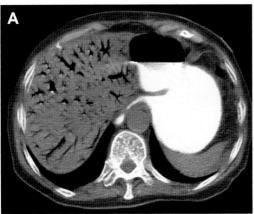 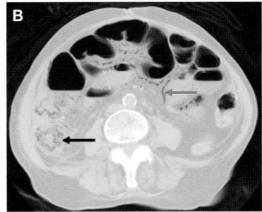

Fig. 21. Colon and small bowel infarction associated with portal venous gas: MDCT features. (*A*) Scan obtained at the level of the liver demonstrates extensive portal venous gas. (*B*) More caudal scan displayed with lung windows shows small bowel (*red arrow*) and colonic (*black arrow*) pneumatosis.

suspicion. In one series evaluating gastrointestinal complications of cardiac surgery, 11.5% of these gastrointestinal complications were attributable to intestinal ischemia and 1.1% were attributable to mesenteric vascular occlusion. Other complications included upper gastrointestinal hemorrhage (28.6%), gastroesophagitis (12.2%), colitis (12.2%), pancreatitis (8.8%), cholecystitis (6.8%), perforated peptic ulcer (4.7%), diverticulitis (3.4%), and lower gastrointestinal hemorrhage (0.7%).[17]

Prognosis

It is important to differentiate the cause of AMI because of variation in disease progression, response to treatment, and outcome. The prognosis is better after acute MVT than that after acute

arterial MI. The prognosis after mesenteric arterial embolism is better than that after arterial thrombosis or nonocclusive ischemia. The mortality rate after surgical treatment of arterial embolism and venous thrombosis (54.1% and 32.1%, respectively) is less than that after surgery for arterial thrombosis and nonocclusive ischemia (77.4% and 72.7%, respectively).[10]

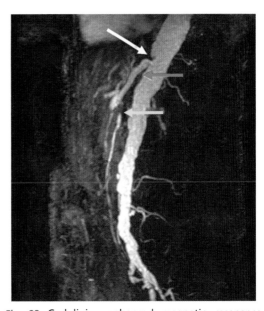

Fig. 23. Gadolinium-enhanced magnetic resonance angiogram in an elderly man with intestinal angina. Sagittal image shows marked atherosclerotic disease of the abdominal aorta and stenosis (*white arrow*) of the origin of the celiac artery. The proximal portion of the SMA is completely occluded (*red arrow*) and reconstitutes distally (*yellow arrow*) by means of collaterals from the celiac artery.

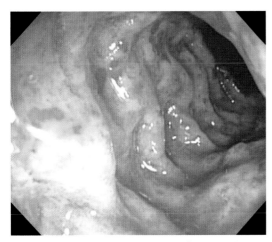

Fig. 22. Ischemic colitis: colonoscopic findings. There is hemorrhage, edema, and an almost a bluish appearance of the colon wall in this patient who has severe ischemic colitis.

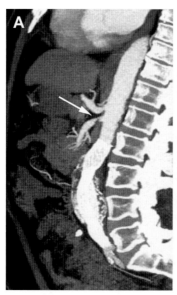
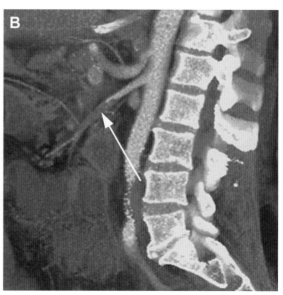

Fig. 24. SMA emboli. (*A*) Sagittal reformatted maximum intensity projection (MIP) MDCT image demonstrates a small embolism (*arrow*) in the SMA. (*B*) In a different patient, a larger embolism (*arrow*) is seen in a more distal portion of the SMA.

DIAGNOSTIC IMAGING MODALITIES
Plain Abdominal Radiographs

Most patients who have intestinal ischemia demonstrate nonspecific findings, such as intestinal dilatation (see **Fig. 12**), gasless abdomen, a small bowel pseudo-obstruction pattern, or paralytic

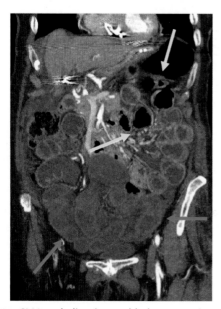

Fig. 25. SMA embolism in an elderly woman in septic shock. Coronal reformatted MDCT shows diminished enhancement of the ileum (*red arrows*) in comparison to the jejunum (*yellow arrows*).

ileus. More specific but far less common findings include thumbprinting in which multiple, round, smooth soft tissue densities project into the intestinal lumen because of mucosal and submucosal edema and hemorrhage. Specific late signs indicating infarction include pneumatosis intestinalis (PI; see **Fig. 13**) and portal venous gas. In most cases of patients who have intestinal ischemia, however, plain radiographs are of limited value.[27–39]

Barium Studies

Barium studies have been replaced by MDCT and, to a lesser degree, MR imaging and ultrasound in the clinical setting of acute intestinal ischemia. Like plain abdominal radiographs, barium studies are too nonspecific and insensitive in evaluating the mural, mesenteric, and vascular manifestations of ischemia. Furthermore, dense barium interferes with subsequent MDCT examinations and transcatheter interventions.Colonoscopy is the most accurate means of establishing the diagnosis of ischemic colitis (**Fig. 22**).

Barium studies still are of some value in the setting of chronic intestinal angina and radiation enteritis. The hallmark of small bowel ischemia on conventional barium studies is thickening of the valvulae conniventes and "thumbprinting." The intramural accumulation of blood may distend the submucosa to such a degree that the folds become focally dilated and flattened, especially along the mesenteric border of the bowel.[19,40,41]

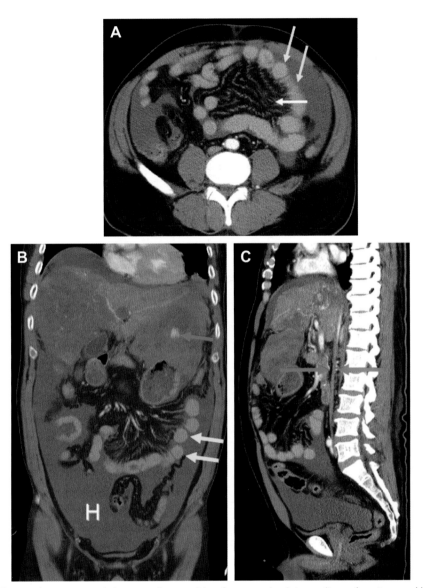

Fig. 26. NOMI secondary to systemic hypotension resulting from massive intraperitoneal rupture and hemorrhage of hepatocellular carcinoma of the left lobe of the liver. (A) Axial MDCT scan shows a hyperdense bowel (*yellow arrows*) secondary to intramural and mucosal hemorrhage. Note the patent vasa rectae (*white arrow*) and hemoperitoneum. (B) Coronal reformatted MDCT image shows the massive hemoperitoneum (H), the hyperdense small bowel (*yellow arrows*), and active extravasation of contrast material in the left hepatic lobe neoplasm (*red arrow*). (C) Sagittal reformatted MDCT image shows a slit-like inferior vena cava (*red arrows*), attesting to the compromised cardiovascular status of the patient.

Angiography

Before the late 1990s and the introduction of MDCT, catheter angiography was the reference standard for the diagnosis of intestinal ischemia.[23,42,43] This is an invasive procedure that has now been supplanted by CT angiography (CTA) and magnetic resonance angiography (MRA).[44] Angiography is now primarily performed immediately before transcatheter intervention.

Transcatheter therapy is currently the intervention of choice in patients who have chronic intestinal angina. This involves the placement of a stent usually in the SMA (see **Fig. 16**). If there is high-grade stenosis (>70%) of the celiac trunk and SMA, both vessels are stented if technically feasible.[45]

Doppler Ultrasound

Because of its dependence on patient factors, including body habitus, the presence of air-filled

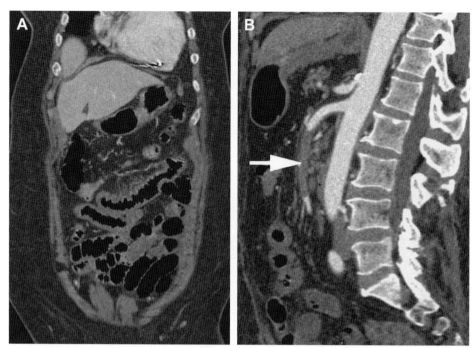

Fig. 27. SMA thrombosis. (*A*) Coronal MPR demonstrates minimal to moderate mural thickening of multiple small bowel loops in the midabdomen. The wall is homogeneous in attenuation. (*B*) Sagittal MPR demonstrates thrombus (*arrow*) in the SMA. There is narrowing and calcification of the origin of the celiac artery, which is probably related to chronic atherosclerotic disease. (*From* Horton KM, Fishman EK. Vascular disorders of the small bowel. In: Gore RM, Levine MS, editors. Textbook of gastrointestinal radiology. 3rd edition. Philadelphia: WB Saunders; 2008. p. 905; with permission.)

bowel loops, prior operations, and patient cooperation, ultrasound is not typically used in the initial evaluation of acutely ill patients who are suspected of having acute intestinal ischemia.[46–50]

In patients who have chronic intestinal angina, Doppler ultrasound can be useful in the detection of celiac artery and SMA stenoses. Peak systolic velocity of greater than 275 cm/s in the SMA and 200 cm/s in the celiac artery indicates greater than 70% stenosis of these vessels (see **Fig. 16**).[34–36]

MR Imaging

MR imaging and MRA can be used to image the gut, mesentery, and surrounding vasculature directly.[51–54] MR imaging, however, is best used in the nonacute setting. The critically ill patient who is suspected of having intestinal ischemia typically has a life support apparatus incompatible with the MR imaging scanner. These patients are best scanned with MDCT, which also offers better spatial resolution.[55,56] The theoretic advantage of using gadolinium-based intravascular contrast agents for MR imaging and MRA rather than the iodinated contrast used in CT in patients with renal insufficiency has been negated by the increasing

incidence of nephrogenic systemic fibrosis related to the gadolinium-based MR imaging contrast agents.

In patients who have chronic intestinal angina, contrast enhanced three-dimensional MRA (**Fig. 23**) provides anatomic information similar to conventional angiography, and its effectiveness in evaluating the mesenteric circulation has been well documented.[57]

Multidetector CT

MDCT has become the preferred imaging technique for the evaluation of patients who are suspected of having acute and chronic intestinal ischemia. It can be performed quickly in critically ill patients and depends less on operator skill and patient factors than other imaging examinations.[30,58–63]

MDCT produces a volume data set that can be reformatted and viewed in any projection, affording exquisite visualization of the bowel wall, surrounding fat, mesenteries, and omenta, which may all show abnormalities with ischemia or infarction. CTA can visualize even tiny distal vascular segments and depict stenoses and their causes: atherosclerotic plaque, thrombus,

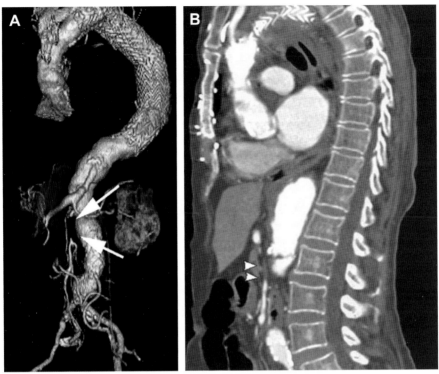

Fig. 28. Occlusive thrombus of the SMA. (A) Volume rendering shows a defect in the SMA (*arrows*). Note the thoracic aorta stent graft. (B) Sagittal reformatted image better demonstrates the thrombus (*arrowheads*).

anatomic abnormalities (eg, obstruction), and tumor.[18,25,59,64–78]

ACUTE ARTERIAL AND VENOUS MESENTERIC ISCHEMIA

The clinical setting of AMI is characterized by the combination of a difficult diagnosis, high fatality rates, and the need for rapid and aggressive diagnostic and therapeutic interventions in patients who are often elderly and have multiple comorbidities.[26]

There are four main categories of AMI: SMAE (50%), NOMI (20%–30%), SMAT (15%–25%), and superior mesenteric vein thrombosis (SMVT) (5%).[1–3]

Superior Mesenteric Artery Embolism (SMAE)

The wide caliber and narrow takeoff angle of the SMA off the aorta make it particularly vulnerable to embolic events. The offending emboli (**Figs. 24 and 25**) usually originate from a left atrial or ventricular mural thrombus or vegetations on a heart valve. Nearly one half of patients who have SMAT have synchronous extramesenteric emboli, including peripheral artery emboli, and 20% have synchronous emboli to the spleen, kidneys, or other organs.[79]

The embolism usually lodges in the proximal SMA, 3 to 10 cm from its origin, in a tapered segment just distal to the middle colic artery branch, although some 15% of emboli cause occlusion at the origin of the SMA. Multiple emboli are present in 20% of cases.[17] Emboli that occur proximal to the origin of the ileocolic artery are considered "major"; "minor" emboli are those that lodge in the SMA distal to the takeoff of the ileocolic artery or in the distal branches of the SMA.[8]

Nonocclusive Mesenteric Ischemia (NOMI)

The diagnosis of NOMI is made by excluding other causes of intestinal ischemia, such as atherosclerosis, arterial or venous thrombosis, embolism, or vasculitis. NOMI is seen in the setting of splanchnic vasoconstriction precipitated by hypoperfusion from acute myocardial infarction, congestive heart failure, arrhythmias, shock (**Fig. 26**), cirrhosis, sepsis, hypovolemia, chronic renal disease, medications, and the use of splanchnic vasoconstrictors.[1,2]

The angiographic features of NOMI include (1) narrowing of the origins of the SMA branches, (2) irregularities of these branches, (3) spasm of the mesenteric arcades, and (4) impaired filling of the intramural vessels.[2,23]

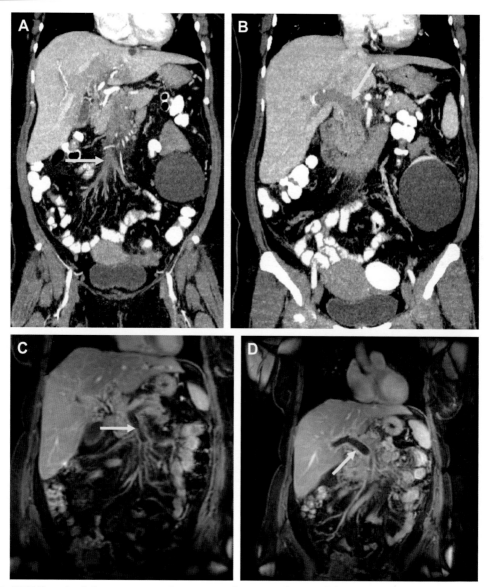

Fig. 29. SMV thrombosis in a woman on hormone replacement therapy. (*A*) Coronal reformatted MDCT images show thrombus (*yellow arrow*) in the first- and second-order tributaries of the SMV. (*B*) Thrombus (*yellow arrow*) is present in the main portal vein. There is mural thickening of the duodenum with some stranding of the adjacent fat, but most of the small bowel and right colon appear remarkably normal. Coronal MR imaging shows thrombus in the SMV (*yellow arrow*) (*C*) and main portal vein (*yellow arrow*) (*D*).

Shock bowel is a subtype of NOMI and is caused by prolonged hypoperfusion because of hypovolemic shock.[80,81] This is a transient phenomenon that resolves with restoration of normotension. Shock bowel causes increased permeability of the bowel wall to macromolecules, and the mural thickening and intraluminal fluid are attributable to failure of fluid resorption.

MDCT shows diffuse abnormalities of the small intestine, including mural and mucosal thickening, dilation, increased luminal fluid, lumen dilation, increased mural enhancement, and a normal-appearing colon.[29] There is a decreased caliber of the abdominal aorta and inferior vena cava and moderate to large peritoneal fluid collections. The mural changes are attributable to increased mucosal permeability related to oxygen hypoperfusion, failed resorption capacity, slow flow, and interstitial leakage of contrast material. This appearance should be distinguished from the diffuse small bowel mural edema that accompanies aggressive volume resuscitation in the setting of trauma.

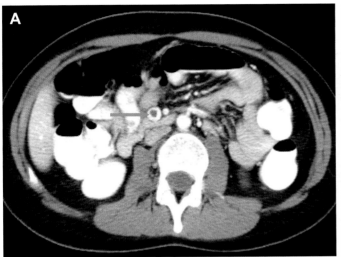
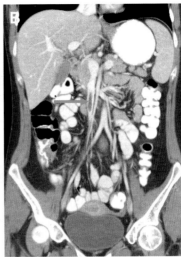

Fig. 30. SMVT in a patient who has Leiden factor V deficiency who presented with nondescript abdominal pain. The coagulopathy was discovered after this scan prompted a hematologic workup. Axial (A) and coronal (B) reformatted MDCT images show a long clot (red arrow) in the SMV without significant intestinal or mesenteric ischemic change.

These patients show signs of elevated central venous pressure that include periportal edema, a dilated inferior vena cava, increased attenuation of mesenteric and retroperitoneal fat, and normal mural enhancement of the small bowel.[31,80,81]

Superior Mesenteric Artery Thrombosis (SMAT)

Because of previously developed collateral vessels, SMAT (Figs. 27 and 28) may have a somewhat more insidious onset than SMAE. The acute ischemic event is commonly superimposed on CMI and 20% to 50% of these patients have a history of postprandial abdominal pain, food aversion, and weight loss during the weeks to months before the seminal event. Because of the antecedent stenosing atherosclerosis, patients who have SMAT usually tend to develop symptoms more subacutely than those patients who have SMAE.[17,18]

Superior Mesenteric Vein Thrombosis (SMVT)

MVT (Figs. 29–31) occurs as an acute, subacute (weeks to months), or chronic disorder. The mean age of these patients is 48 to 60 years, which is younger than those with other forms of AMI. As many as 60% of patients have a history of peripheral vein thrombosis.[2,8]

The location of the primary thrombus within the mesenteric venous circulation depends on the cause. MVT attributable to cirrhosis, neoplasm, or operative injury begins at the site of obstruction and propagates peripherally. Thrombosis

attributable to hypercoagulable states starts in smaller branches and propagates into the major trunks. MVT is associated with an extremely wide clinical spectrum ranging from a relatively asymptomatic patient in whom the thrombosis is diagnosed incidentally to an acute, severe, life-threatening disease.[1–4,8]

The degree of thrombosis may be large, but intestinal infarction is rare unless the branches of the peripheral arcades and the vasa recta are involved. If the collateral circulation is inadequate and venous drainage from the involved segment is compromised, the affected intestine becomes congested, edematous, cyanotic, and thickened with intramural hemorrhage.[1] Serosanguineous peritoneal fluid heralds early hemorrhagic infarction.[8]

CHRONIC MESENTERIC ISCHEMIA

Atherosclerosis of the mesenteric circulation is quite common, particularly in the elderly population. Symptomatic CMI, however, is rare because of the development of extensive collaterals. Risk factors for the development of CMI include a positive family history, smoking, hypertension, and hypercholesterolemia, the same risk factors as for atherosclerosis. There is a female predominance of symptomatic disease.

Nonatherosclerotic causes of CMI are less frequent and include celiac artery compression (median arcuate ligament syndrome), chronic aortic dissection, inflammatory arterial disease, aortic coarctation, middle aortic syndrome, fibromuscular dysplasia, and neurofibromatosis.

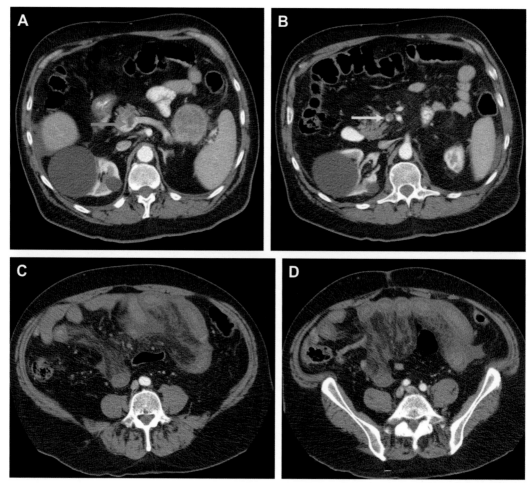

Fig. 31. SMVT: MDCT findings. (*A*) Thrombus (*red arrow*) is identified at the confluence of the SMA and splenic veins. Thrombus is present in both vessels. (*B*) Scan obtained at a slightly more caudal level shows almost complete occlusion of the SMV (*yellow arrow*). (*C, D*) Scans obtained more caudally show mural thickening of the involved loops with submucosal edema, mural hemorrhage, mesenteric edema, and hemorrhage.

COLONIC ISCHEMIA

CI is the most common vascular disorder of the gut in elderly patients. The colon is predisposed to ischemia because of the fact that it receives less blood flow per gram of tissue than does the remainder of the gastrointestinal tract.[28,29] Indeed, there is an extensive network of intramural vessels arising from the vasa recta and vasa brevia in the mesenteric border of the gut that gives rise to a microvascular plexus in the muscularis propria and submucosal layer and is less well developed in the colon compared with the thinner walled small bowel.[1,2]

CI encompasses a spectrum of injury that may be reversible or irreversible. CI can be further categorized as (1) reversible ischemic colonopathy (submucosal or intramural hemorrhage), (2) reversible or transient ischemic colitis, (3) chronic ulcerative ischemic colitis, (4) ischemic colonic stricture, (5) colonic gangrene, and (6) fulminant universal ischemic colitis. Many cases of transient or reversible ischemia of the colon are missed because the disease is self-limited.[24]

PNEUMATOSIS INTESTINALIS

Intramural gas is associated with several disorders ranging from life-threatening to benign.[82] PI pathogenically derives from four major categories: bowel necrosis, mucosal disruption, increased mucosal permeability, and pulmonary disease.[83] The first three causes may be found in patients who have intestinal ischemia (see **Figs. 13–15, 20,** and **21**). In patients who have intestinal ischemia, gas may dissect from the intestinal lumen because of an increase in intraluminal pressure (eg, from obstruction) or mucosal compromise (eg, ischemia, infarction). At the same time, gas-forming bacilli enter the submucosa through mucosal rents and produce intramural gas.[82–84]

In the presence of PI in the setting of suspected intestinal ischemia, PI and the following elevated markers are associated with a poor prognosis: acidosis with a blood pH less than 7.3, hyperamylasemia of greater than 200 IU/L, a serum bicarbonate level of less than 20 mmol/L, and an elevated serum lactic acid level of greater than 2 mmol/L. Indeed, the presence of lactic acidosis greater than 2 mmol/L in patients who had PI was associated with a greater than 80% mortality rate.[84]

PI is useful in differentiating early and nontransmural MI from full-thickness and irreversible transmural infarction. Linear PI is more often seen than bubbly PI in patients who have transmural bowel infarction. PI that accompanies portomesenteric venous gas correlates strongly with transmural bowel infarction, whereas PI without evidence of portomesenteric gas may have a more benign course.[39,60,76]

FOCAL SEGMENTAL MESENTERIC ISCHEMIA

Short-segment ischemic disease may be caused by a large number of disorders, including vasculitis, medications, surgery, radiation, neoplasm, and, most importantly, bowel obstruction. Most cases of localized MI show similar radiologic features. It is important, however, to determine the underlying cause to guide diagnostic and therapeutic planning. The clinical presentation of localized MI depends on the length and distribution of the ischemia and the course of disease.[30,33]

With the exception of strangulated bowel obstruction, there is usually adequate collateral circulation to prevent transmural hemorrhagic infarction; however, the affected bowel often becomes secondarily infected. Limited tissue necrosis may go on to complete healing, chronic enteritis, or stricture formation.[30]

Bowel Obstruction

Strangulation and infarction (**Figs. 32** and **33**) are the most dreaded complications of bowel obstruction. Strangulation is usually seen in the setting of a closed-loop obstruction caused by volvulus, adhesions and bands, and internal or external hernias. This complication occurs in approximately 10% of patients who have small bowel obstruction and carries a high mortality rate of 20% to 37%.[36]

The mural changes associated with closed-loop obstruction and strangulation include circumferential mural thickening (>3 mm), the target or halo sign (indicating submucosal edema), focal

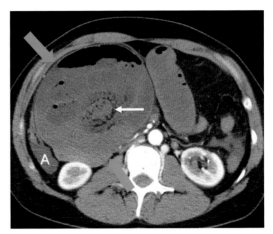

Fig. 32. Right paraduodenal internal hernia associated with bowel obstruction and ischemia. Note the poor enhancement of the obstructed loops (*red arrows*), increased intraluminal secretions, and swirling of the mesentery (*white arrow*). A, ascites.

loss of mural enhancement (impaired arterial flow), persistent mural enhancement (impaired venous outflow), mural hemorrhage or haziness on noncontrast scans, and pneumatosis.[30,36]

The mesenteric changes associated with closed-loop obstruction include radial configuration of bowel loops when vertically oriented; convergence of mesenteric vessels to a single point; close proximity of afferent and efferent limbs, often at the site of mesenteric convergence; a beak or whirl sign at the point of obstruction; C-shaped, U-shaped, or coffee bean configuration of the bowel loop with convergence toward the torsion; engorged mesenteric veins; mesenteric stranding or hemorrhage; ascites; portomesenteric venous gas; and perforation.[20,30,36]

Neoplasms

Ischemic colitis is a well-recognized complication of obstructing colon carcinoma, developing in some 1% to 7% of cases.[85] The bowel distention and elevated intraluminal pressure caused by the cancer produce vascular impairment in the mucosa and submucosa, leading to mucosal damage identical to ischemic colitis. The integrity of the colonic wall is further compromised by stagnation of fecal material above the tumor and by mechanical occlusion resulting from recurrent transient colonic twisting or torsion produced by the cancer.

It is important to recognize ischemia proximal to colon cancer for two reasons. First, ischemia imperils a primary colonic anastomotic suture line, and postoperative complications occur in up to 25% of proximal ischemic colitis cases.[30,86]

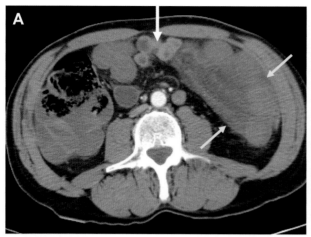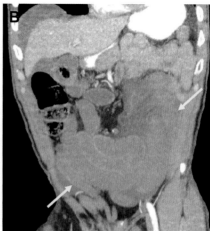

Fig. 33. Closed-loop obstruction causing small bowel infarction. (*A*) CT scan shows cluster (*white arrow*) of closely opposed narrowed segments of small bowel. Note the mural thickening of obstructed loops with hemorrhage in the adjacent small bowel mesentery (*yellow arrows*). (*B*) Coronal reformatted image clearly depicts the hypoenhancement of the small bowel loops within the closed-loop obstruction. Ascites is also present.

Second, ischemic colitis may lead to secondary congestive changes in the pericolic or perirectal fat that can simulate T3 invasion, leading to overstaging of tumor on CT.[59,70,87] Similarly, the mural thickening that accompanies the ischemia may give a false impression of the length of tumor involvement, which can have important therapeutic implications in rectal cancers. One useful differentiating feature on CT is the fact that the mural thickening associated with ischemia causes submucosal edema, which leads to preservation of mural stratification and the so-called "target" sign. Colonic wall thickened by tumor is inhomogeneous in attenuation with loss of mural stratification.[30,81] When a right-sided colon cancer obstructs the ileocecal valve, the resultant increased intraluminal pressure within the small bowel may lead to small intestinal ischemia.[30,81]

Drug Induced Enterocolitis

A wide variety of orally and parenterally administered medications can cause small bowel ischemia and CI. Estrogens and oral contraceptives, which accelerate intravascular coagulation and inhibit fibrinolysis, are major risk factors for the development of thromboembolic events in the mesenteric, portal, and hepatic veins.[1,2]

Several cardiac drugs can have a profound effect on the splanchnic blood supply. Digitalis, inderal, dopamine, and vasopressin are commonly used drugs that can be powerful gut vasoconstrictors; they not only reduce mesenteric blood flow but cause contraction of precapillary sphincters in the intestinal mucosa.[1,2,33]

Chemotherapeutic agents can lead to bowel ischemia and perforation, particularly in patients receiving long-term immunosuppression to prevent homograft rejection and in those patients receiving chemotherapy for leukemia (**Fig. 34**) and lymphoma.[10,11,33]

Radiation Enterocolitis

Endarteritis obliterans is the microvascular lesion that develops in patients who receive abdominopelvic radiation therapy at doses of 45 to 60 Gy. The sigmoid colon, rectum, and terminal ileum (**Fig. 35**) are the sites most commonly affected by this progressive occlusive vasculitis that can lead to bowel ischemia, infarction, perforation, bleeding, and stricture and fistula formation.[33] Risk factors that predispose to the development of chronic radiation enteritis include hypertension, atherosclerosis, diabetes, prior abdominal surgery with adhesions, and a history of peritonitis.[32]

The diagnosis of radiation enterocolitis is difficult, because the latent period between the radiation therapy and the development of radiation damage is usually 6 to 24 months but can be longer than 20 years. It may simulate clinically and radiologically recurrent cancer or adhesive disease.[1,2]

Trauma

Trauma is an important cause of intestinal ischemia. Blunt trauma, especially attributable to motor vehicle collisions, can lead to seat-belt injury to the intestine and mesentery. The small bowel and its mesentery can be crushed between the seat belt and spine, causing a hematoma, transverse tear

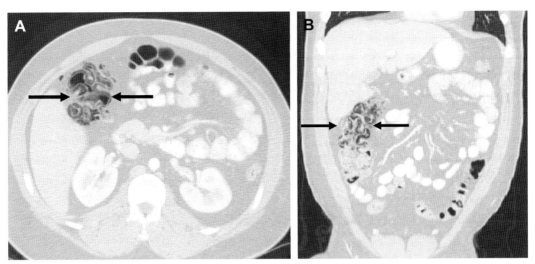

Fig. 34. CI in an immunocompromised patient receiving chemotherapy for acute myelogenous leukemia. Pneumatosis (*arrows*) of the right colon is identified on these axial (*A*) and coronal (*B*) MDCT images displayed with lung windows.

of the mesentery, and, ultimately, small bowel ischemia and infarction. The mesenteric tear interferes with local blood supply, and the resultant ischemia can be difficult to differentiate from non-ischemic mural thickening attributable to contusion. Additionally, the rapid deceleration can cause jejunal transection at a site within 20 cm of the ligament of Treitz, because the shearing force is directed between the relatively fixed proximal and more mobile distal jejunum.[30,34]

Penetrating trauma can directly injure the aorta, SMA, or IMA, leading to extensive hemoperitoneum or acute intestinal ischemia. If there is

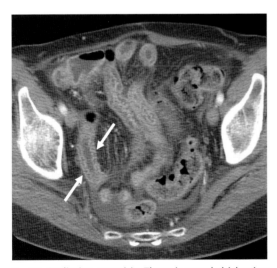

Fig. 35. Radiation enteritis. There is mural thickening (*arrows*) of the terminal ileum in this patient who had received radiation therapy for cervical cancer.

massive blood loss, the mesenteric blood supply to the gut is also compromised, leading to ischemic colitis or, less likely, enteritis, particularly in older individuals with advanced atherosclerotic change.[2]

Vasculitis

When larger vessels are involved, abdominal manifestations of vasculitis involving the mesenteric vessels may be indistinguishable from those of MI caused by emboli or thrombosis, except for associated evidence of systemic disease. Medium-sized arteritis, such as that found in polyarteritis nodosa, has a tendency to form aneurysms that can rupture and lead to intestinal and intraperitoneal hemorrhage.[80]

CT is helpful in differentiating MI caused by vasculitis from that caused by other conditions. Vasculitis preferentially tends to involve the small bowel (**Fig. 36**), whereas thromboembolic disease is more evenly distributed. Vascular thrombosis and atherosclerosis occur more frequently in those patients who have thromboembolic disease, whereas splenomegaly and genitourinary tract disease (eg, nephritis, cystitis, hydronephrosis) are more common in the vasculitis group.[80] Accordingly, vasculitis should be suspected as the cause of MI in a younger patient; in those patients who have synchronous disease of the stomach, duodenum, or rectum; or when these is concomitant involvement of the small bowel and large bowel.[30,80]

In patients who have polyarteritis nodosa, the pattern of bowel ischemia is usually multifocal and nonsegmental with long segments of bowel

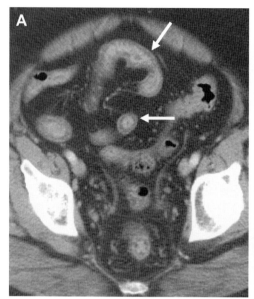 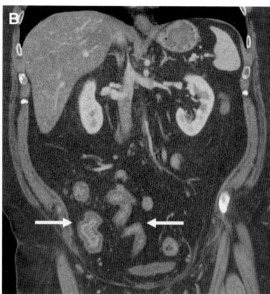

Fig. 36. Lupus vasculitis. Several proximal ileal loops demonstrate mural thickening and submucosal edema (*arrows*). These axial (*A*) and coronal (*B*) reformatted images also show edema in the mesentery.

involvement. Primary duodenal involvement points to vasculitis as well.[79,80]

THERAPEUTIC OPTIONS

Patients who are suspected of having AMI require volume resuscitation; correction of hypotension, congestive heart failure, and cardiac arrhythmias; correction of acid-base and electrolyte abnormalities; and infusion of broad-spectrum antibiotics offering theoretic protection against the bacterial translocation that accompanies loss of mural integrity.[26] Specific therapies are discussed next.

Superior Mesenteric Artery Embolism

Infusion of vasodilators (papaverine) and thrombolytic agents (eg, streptokinase, urokinase, recombinant tissue plasminogen activator) is useful in patients without signs of peritonitis.[5] Embolism in the SMA induces a profound vasoconstriction of obstructed and nonobstructed branches of the SMA. If not promptly corrected, this vasoconstriction can become irreversible and persist even after the surgical removal of the embolus. Thrombolytic therapy is most likely to be successful when the thrombus is minor (distal to the origin of the ileocolic artery), when it is given within 12 hours of the onset of symptoms, and when the thrombus is only partially occluding.[2] When signs of peritonitis are present, laparotomy is indicated with the intent to restore intestinal blood flow and resect necrotic bowel.[7]

Superior Mesenteric Artery Thrombosis

The treatment of choice is emergency surgical revascularization with continuous preoperative papaverine. Thrombolysis and angioplasty have also been used in this clinical setting.[10]

Nonocclusive Mesenteric Ischemia

In accordance[26] with the pathophysiology of this disorder, there are two major principles of treatment: (1) correction of predisposing and precipitating factors and (2) treatment of the mesenteric vasoconstriction. In the absence of sepsis or peritoneal signs, vasodilator therapy is used. Patients are referred to laparotomy when there is no reaction to vasodilator infusion or if serum markers suggest necrosis or peritonitis.[17] Infusional agents include papaverine, prostaglandin E_1, phenoxybenzamine, tolazoline, and laevodosine.[2,19]

Chronic Mesenteric Ischemia (Intestinal Agina)

Percutaneous therapy is currently the therapy of choice and can also be used in critically ill patients. This involves the placement of a stent, usually in the SMA. If there is high-grade stenosis (>70%) of the celiac trunk and SMA, both vessels should be stented if technically feasible.[12]

Superior Mesenteric Venous Thrombosis

In asymptomatic patients in whom SMVT is diagnosed, a 3- to 6-month course of anticoagulation may be established. In patients who have symptomatic SMVT, anticoagulation with heparin for 7 to 10 days followed by an oral regimen of Coumadin for 3 to 6 months has been recommended. If peritoneal signs are present, laparotomy with embolectomy is indicated, followed by heparin and papaverine.[1,2,5]

SUMMARY

Gastrointestinal tract ischemia can threaten bowel viability with potentially catastrophic consequences, including intestinal necrosis and gangrene. Because presenting symptoms and signs are relatively nonspecific and imaging findings may be confusing, the diagnosis of intestinal tract ischemia requires a high index of suspicion. It is important to attempt to determine the cause of the intestinal ischemia and differentiate between intestinal ischemia and infarction. The early inclusion of bowel ischemia and infarction in the differential diagnosis of patients with abdominal pain accompanied by an aggressive diagnostic and therapeutic approach may be the only way to improve patient survival in this potentially lethal disorder.

REFERENCES

1. Brandt LJ. Intestinal ischemia. In: Feldman M, Friedman LS, Brandt LJ, editors. Gastrointestinal and liver disease. 8th edition. Philadelphia: Saunders; 2006. p. 2563–88.
2. Burns BJ, Brandt JL. Intestinal ischemia. Gastroenterol Clin North Am 2003;32:1127–43.
3. Yasuhara H. Acute mesenteric ischemia: the challenge of gastroenterology. Surg Today 2005;35:185–95.
4. Chang JG, Stein TA. Mesenteric ischemia: acute and chronic. Ann Vasc Surg 2003;17:323–8.
5. Haglund U, Bergqvist D. Intestinal ischemia—the basics. Langenbecks Arch Surg 1999;384:233–8.
6. Martinez JP, Hogan GJ. Mesenteric ischemia. Emerg Med Clin North Am 2004;22:909–28.
7. Kolkman JJ, Mensink PB, van Petersen AS, et al. Clinical approach to chronic gastrointestinal ischaemia: from "intestinal angina" to the spectrum of chronic splanchnic disease. Scand J Gastroenterol Suppl 2004;241(Suppl):9–16.
8. Clavien PA, Durig M, Harder F. Venous mesenteric infarction: a particular entity. Br J Surg 1988;75:252–8.
9. Korotinski S, Katz A, Malnick SD. Chronic ischaemic bowel diseases in the aged—go with the flow. Age Ageing 2005;34:10–6.
10. Schoots IG, Koffeman GI, Legemate DA, et al. Systemic review of survival after acute mesenteric ischemia according to disease aetiology. Br J Surg 2004;91:17–27.
11. Van Bockel JH, Geelkerken RH, Wasser MN. Chronic splanchnic ischaemia. Best Pract Res Clin Gastroenterol. 2001;15(1):99–119.
12. Comerota AJ, Miller MT. Mesenteric ischemia. In: Yeo CJ, Dempsey DT, Klein AS, et al, editors. Surgery of the alimentary tract. 6th edition. Philadelphia: Saunders; 2005. p. 1247–64.
13. Tendler DA. Acute intestinal ischemia and infarction. Semin Gastrointest Dis 2003;14:66–76.
14. Hart J. Non-neoplastic diseases of the small and large intestine. In: Silverberg SG, editor. Surgical pathology and cytopathology. 4th edition. New York: Churchill-Livingston; 2006. p. 467–85.
15. Rosai J. Gastrointestinal tract. In: Rosai J, editor. Surgical pathology. 9th edition. Edinburgh (UK): Mosby; 2004. p. 615–872.
16. Goldin SB, Rosemurgy A. Anatomy and physiology of the mesenteric circulation. In: Yeo CJ, Dempsey DT, Klein AS, et al, editors. Surgery of the alimentary tract. 6th edition. Philadelphia: Saunders; 2005. p. 1235–46.
17. Ujiki M, Kibbe MR. Mesenteric ischemia. Perspect Vasc Surg Endovasc Ther 2005;17:309–18.
18. Sreenarasimhaiah J. Diagnosis and management of intestinal ischaemic disorders. BMJ 2003;326:1372–6.
19. Trompeter M, Brazda T, Remy CT, et al. Non-occlusive mesenteric ischemia: etiology, diagnosis, and interventional therapy. Eur Radiol 2002;12:1179–87.
20. Chang RW, Chang JB, Longo WE. Update in management of mesenteric ischemia. World J Gastroenterol 2006;12:3243–7.
21. Sreenarasimhaiah J. Chronic mesenteric ischaemia. Best Pract Res Clin Gastroenterol 2005;19(2):283–95.
22. Ruotolo RA, Evans SR. Mesenteric ischemia in the elderly. Clin Geriatr Med 1999;15:527–57.
23. Bakal C, Sprayregen S, Wolf E. Radiology in intestinal ischemia: angiographic diagnosis and management. Surg Clin North Am 1992;72:125–32.
24. Greenwald DA, Brandt LJ, Reinus JF. Ischemic bowel disease in the elderly. Gastroenterol Clin North Am 2001;30:445–73.
25. Liolios A, Oropello JM, Benjamin E. Gastrointestinal complications in the intensive care unit. Clin Chest Med 1999;20:329–45.
26. Lock G. Acute intestinal ischaemia. Best Pract Res Clin Gastroenterol 2001;15(1):83–98.
27. Romano S, Lassandro F, Scaglione M, et al. Ischemia and infarction of the small bowel and colon: spectrum of imaging findings. Abdom Imaging. 2006;31:277–92.
28. Romano S, Romano L, Grassi R. Multidetector row computed tomography findings from ischemia to

infarction of the large bowel. Eur J Radiol 2007;61: 433–41.

29. Mirvis SE, Shanmuganathan K, Erb R. Diffuse small-bowel ischemia in hypotensive adults after blunt trauma (shock bowel): CT findings and clinical significance. AJR Am J Roentgenol 194;163:1375–1379.

30. Kim AY, Ha HK. Evaluation of suspected mesenteric ischemia: efficacy of radiologic studies. Radiol Clin North Am 2003;41:327–42.

31. Shanmuganathan K, Mirvis SE, Amorosa M. Periportal low density on CT in patients with blunt trauma: association with elevated venous pressure. AJR Am J Roentgenol 1993;160:279–83.

32. Rha SE, Ha HK, Lee S-H, et al. CT and MR imaging findings of bowel ischemia from various primary causes. Radiographics 2000;20:29–42.

33. Ha HK, Rha SE, Kim AY, et al. CT and MR diagnoses of intestinal ischemia. Semin Ultrasound CT MR 2000;21:40–55.

34. Halvorsen RA, Camacho MA. Abdominal trauma. In: Gore RM, Levine MS, editors. Textbook of gastrointestinal radiology. 3rd edition. Philadelphia: Saunders; 2008. p. 2417–37.

35. Gore RM, Szucs RA, Wolf EL, et al. Miscellaneous abnormalities of the colon. In: Gore RM, Levine MS, editors. Textbook of gastrointestinal radiology. 3rd edition. Philadelphia: Saunders; 2008. p. 1203–34.

36. Gore RM, Yaghmai V, Mehta V, et al. The acute abdomen. In: Gore RM, Levine MS, editors. Textbook of gastrointestinal radiology. 3rd edition. Philadelphia: Saunders; 2008. p. 2385–403.

37. Baker SR, Cho KC. The abdominal plain film with correlative imaging. 2nd edition. Appleton & Lange: Stamford (CT); 1999. p. 315–29.

38. Messmer JM. Gas and soft tissue abnormalities. In: Gore RM, Levine MS, editors. Textbook of gastrointestinal radiology. 3rd edition. The acute abdomen. Philadelphia: Saunders; 2008. p. 205–24.

39. Smerud MJ, Johnson CD, Stephens DH. Diagnosis of bowel infarction: a comparison of plain films and CT scans in 23 cases. AJR Am J Roentgenol 1990; 154:99–103.

40. Wolf EJ, Sprayregen S, Bakal CW. Radiology in intestinal ischemia. Plain film, contrast, and other imaging studies. Surg Clin North Am 1992;72: 107–24.

41. Rubesin SE. Miscellaneous abnormalities of the small bowel. In: Gore RM, Levine MS, editors. Textbook of gastrointestinal radiology. 3rd edition. Philadelphia: Saunders; 2008. p. 933–43.

42. Kim ST, Nemcek AA, Vogelzang RL. Angiography and interventional radiology of the hollow viscera. In: Gore RM, Levine MS, editors. Textbook of gastrointestinal radiology. 3rd edition. Philadelphia: Saunders; 2008. p. 117–40.

43. Klein HM, Lensing R, Klosterhalfen B, et al. Diagnostic imaging of mesenteric infarction. Radiology 1995; 197:79–82.

44. Piffaretti G, Tozzi M, Lomazzi C, et al. Endovascular therapy for chronic mesenteric ischemia. World J Surg. 2007;31:2416–21.

45. Sarac TP, Altinel O, Kashyap V, et al. Endovascular treatment of stenotic and occluded visceral arteries for chronic mesenteric ischemia. J Vasc Surg. 2008; 47:485–91.

46. Dietrich CF, Jedrzejczyk M, Ignee A. Sonographic assessment of the splanchnic arteries and the bowel wall. Eur J Radiol 2007;64:202–12.

47. Zwolak RM, Fillinger MF, Walsh DB, et al. Mesenteric and celiac duplex scanning: a validation study. J Vasc Surg 1998;27:1078–87.

48. Hamada T, Yamauchi M, Tanaka M, et al. Prospective evaluation of contrast-enhanced ultrasonography with advanced dynamic flow for the diagnosis of intestinal ischaemia. Br J Radiol. 2007;80:603–8.

49. Armstrong PA. Visceral duplex scanning: evaluation before and after artery intervention for chronic mesenteric ischemia. Perspect Vasc Surg Endovasc Ther. 2007;19:386–92.

50. Mitchell EL. Moneta GL. Mesenteric duplex scanning. Perspect Vasc Surg Endovasc Ther. 2006;18: 175–83.

51. Meany JF. Non-invasive evaluation of the visceral arteries with magnetic resonance angiography. Eur Radiol 1999;9:1267–76.

52. Gaa J, Laub G, Edelman RR, et al. First clinical results of ultrafast, contrast-enhanced 2-phase 3D magnetic resonance angiography technique for imaging visceral abdominal arteries and veins. Invest Radiol 2000;35:111–7.

53. Shirkoda A, Konez O, Shetty AN, et al. Mesenteric circulation: three-dimensional MR angiography with a gadolinium-enhanced multiecho gradient-echo technique. Radiology 1997;202:257–61.

54. Michaely HJ, Attenberger UI, Kramer H, et al. Abdominal and pelvic MR angiography. Magn Reson Imaging Clin N Am 2007;15:301–14.

55. Michaely HJ, Dietrich O, Nael K, et al. MRA of abdominal vessels: technical advances. Eur Radiol. 2006; 16(8):1637–50.

56. Shih MC, Hagspiel KD. CTA and MRA in mesenteric ischemia: part 1. Role in diagnosis and differential diagnosis. AJR Am J Roentgenol 2007;188(2): 452–61.

57. Shih MC, Angle JF, Leung DA, et al. CTA and MRA in mesenteric ischemia: part 2. Normal findings and complications after surgical and endovascular treatment. AJR Am J Roentgenol. 2007;188(2): 462–71.

58. Van Beers BE, Danse E, Hammer R, et al. Imaging of intestinal ischemia. J Radiol 2004;85:533–8.

59. Segatto E, Mortele KJ, Ji H, et al. Acute bowel ische-mia: CT imaging findings. Semin Ultrasound CT MR 2003;24:364–76.

60. Wiesner W, Khurana B, Ji H, et al. CT of bowel ischemia. Radiology 2003;226:635–50.

61. Horton KM, Fishman EK. Multi-detector row CT of mesenteric ischemia: can it be done? Radio-graphics 2001;21:1463–73.

62. Chou CK, Wu RH, Mak C-W, et al. Clinical signifi-cance of poor CT enhancement of the thickened small-bowel wall in patients with acute abdominal pain. AJR Am J Roentgenol 2006;186:491–8.

63. Wildermuth S, Leschka S, Alkadhi H, et al. Multislice CT in the pre- and postinterventional evaluation of mesen-teric perfusion. Eur Radiol. 2005;15(6):1203–10.

64. Horton KM, Fishman EK. Computed tomography evaluation of intestinal ischemia. Semin Roentgenol 2001;36:118–25.

65. Chou CK, Mak CW, Tzeng WS, et al. CT of small bowel ischemia. Abdom Imaging 2004;29:18–22.

66. Horton KM, Fishman HK. Vascular disorders of the small intestine. In: Gore RM, Levine MS, editors. Textbook of gastrointestinal radiology. 3rd edition. Philadelphia: Saunders; 2008. p. 901–18.

67. Kirkpatrick ID, Kroeker MA, Greenberg HM. Biphasic CT with mesenteric CT angiography in the evaluation of acute mesenteric ischemia: initial experience. Radiology. 2003;229(1):91–8.

68. Horton KM, Fishman EK. Volume-rendered 3D CT of the mesenteric vasculature: normal anatomy, ana-tomic variants, and pathologic conditions. Radio-graphics 2002;22:161–72.

69. Macari M, Balthazar EJ. CT of bowel wall thickening: significance and pitfalls of interpretation. AJR Am J Roentgenol 2001;176:1105–16.

70. Cademartiri F, Raaijmakers RH, Kuiper JW, et al. Multi-detector row CT angiography in patients with abdominal angina. Radiographics 2004;24:969–84.

71. Horton KM, Fishman EK. Multidetector CT angiogra-phy in the diagnosis of mesenteric ischemia. Radiol Clin North Am 2007;45:275–88.

72. Horton KM, Fishman EK. 3D CT angiography of the celiac and superior mesenteric arteries with multide-tector CT data sheets: preliminary observations. Abdom Imaging 2000;25:523–5.

73. Chou CK. CT manifestations of bowel ischemia. AJR Am J Roentgenol 2002;178:87–91.

74. Angelelli G, Scardapane A, Memeo M, et al. Acute bowel ischemia: CT findings. Eur J Radiol 2004;50:37–47.

75. Macari M, Chandarana H, Balthazar E, et al. Intestinal ischemia versus intramural hemorrhage: CT evalua-tion. AJR Am J Roentgenol 2003;180:177–84.

76. Wiesner W, Mortele KJ, Glickman JN, et al. Pneuma-tosis intestinalis and portomesenteric venous gas in intestinal ischemia: correlation of CT findings with severity of ischemia and clinical outcomes. AJR Am J Roentgenol 2001;177:1319–23.

77. Sebastia C, Quiroga S, Epsin E, et al. Porto-mesenteric vein gas: pathologic mechanisms, CT findings, and prognosis. Radiographics 2000;20:1213–24.

78. Ho LN, Paulson EM, Thompson WM. Pneumatosis in the adult: benign to life-threatening causes. AJR Am J Roentgenol 2007;188:1604–13.

79. Lee R, Tung HKS, Tung PHM, et al. CT in acute mesenteric ischaemia. Clin Radiol 2003;58:279–87.

80. Kim JK, Ha HK, Byun JY, et al. CT differentiation of mesenteric ischemia due to vasculitis and thrombo-embolic disease. J Comput Assist Tomogr 2001;25:604–11.

81. Kim AY, Ha HK, Seo BK, et al. CT of patients with right-sided colon cancer and distal ileal thickening. AJR Am J Roentgenol 2000;175:1439–44.

82. Ho LM, Paulson EK, Thompson WM. Pneumatosis intestinalis in the adult: benign to life-threatening causes. AJR Am J Roentgenol 2007;188:1604–13.

83. Pear BL. Pneumatosis intestinalis: a review. Radio-logy 1998;207:13–9.

84. Hawn MT, Canon CL, Lockhart ME, et al. Serum lactic acid determines outcomes of CT diagnosis of pneumatosis of the gastrointestinal tract. Am Surg 2004;70:19–23.

85. Kernagis LY, Levine MS, Jacobs JE. Pneumatosis intestinalis in patients with ischemia: correlation of CT findings with viability of the bowel. AJR Am J Roentgenol 2003;180:733–6.

86. Ko GY, Ha HK, Lee HJ, et al. Usefulness of CT in patients with ischemic colitis proximal to colonic cancer. AJR Am J Roentgenol 1997;168:951–6.

87. Sheedy SP, Earnest F, Fletcher JG, et al. CT of small-bowel ischemia associated with obstruction in emergency department patients: diagnostic perfor-mance evaluation. Radiology 2006;241:729–35.

The Etiology and Pathogenesis of Vascular Disorders of the Intestine

Flavio Paterno, MD[a], Walter E. Longo, MD, FACS, FASCRS[a,b,*]

KEYWORDS

- Mesenteric ischemia • Intestinal ischemia
- Bowel ischemia • Mesenteric infarction • Ischemic colitis

Mesenteric ischemia comprises different clinical syndromes characterized by inadequate blood perfusion to the bowel. It is an important medical condition because of its high mortality rate: Acute mesenteric ischemia is considered a real life-threatening emergency. Intestinal ischemia accounts for 1 of every 1000 hospital admissions and approximately 1 to 2 of every 100 admissions for abdominal pain. Its mortality rates range between 30% and 90% depending on the etiology.[1,2] A Swedish population study based on autopsy (87% autopsy rate) showed that the incidence of acute thromboembolic occlusion of the superior mesenteric artery was 6.8 per 100,000 person years. The estimated overall mortality was 93%. The proportions of cases diagnosed at autopsy only, operation and subsequent autopsy, and operation only, were 65%, 14%, and 21%, respectively. The incidence increased with age, doubling every 5 years up to 217 per 100,000 person years in the age category 85 and above. There was no gender difference when the confounding factor of women predominating in the elderly cohorts was corrected.[3]

HISTORY

Mesenteric ischemia was described for the first time by Antonio Beniviene in Florence in the 15th century. Only in the 19th century, when several investigators reported on this condition, was it finally recognized as clinically relevant. In 1875, Litten performed the first experimental study on the ligature of mesenteric vessels. In 1895, Elliott reported the first successful bowel resection of infarcted intestine. He resected the necrotic bowel leaving two temporary stomas, which he reanastomosed 2 weeks later. The first description of chronic intestinal ischemia was by Councilman in 1894. He reported three patients with chronic occlusion of the superior mesenteric artery (SMA) complaining of abdominal pain. In 1957, Mikkelson introduced the term *intestinal angina* to describe this symptom complex. In 1950, Klass reported the first embolectomy on the SMA with successful reperfusion of the intestine, thus avoiding bowel resection. He described the early presentation of acute mesenteric ischemia with severe abdominal pain, bloody stool, and almost normal physical examination. In 1958, Shaw and Maynard performed the first successful thromboendarterectomy of the SMA for thrombosis. Ende, in 1958, published the first description of nonocclusive mesenteric ischemia (NOMI) associated to cardiac failure, "perhaps aided by vascular spasm," with infarction of the bowel in the absence of mesenteric vascular occlusion. In 1967, Aakhus and Brabrand introduced angiography in the

[a] Yale University School of Medicine, Department of Surgery, 330 Cedar Street, New Haven, CT 06520-8062, USA
[b] Section of Gastrointestinal Surgery, Yale New Haven Hospital, 330 Cedar Street, New Haven, CT 06520-8062, USA
* Corresponding author. Yale University School of Medicine, Department of Surgery, 330 Cedar Street, LH 118, P.O. Box 208062, New Haven, CT 06520-8062.
E-mail address: walter.longo@yale.edu (W.E. Longo).

Radiol Clin N Am 46 (2008) 877–885
doi:10.1016/j.rcl.2008.06.005

diagnostic workup of patients with suspected acute mesenteric ischemia. In 1973, Boley used intra-arterial infusion of papaverine to relieve mesenteric vasoconstriction. Since then, early angiography, papaverine infusion, percutaneous endovascular techniques and early surgery improved the results in the management of acute mesenteric ischemia, lowering the mortality rate to 50% from 80%.[4,5]

ANATOMY

The gastrointestinal tract is perfused by three branches of the abdominal aorta: the celiac trunk, the SMA, and the inferior mesenteric artery (IMA). The celiac axis arises from the aorta at the level of T12. It divides into the left gastric artery, the common hepatic artery, and the splenic artery. It supplies all the upper abdominal viscera, including the stomach, duodenum, spleen, liver, and pancreas. The SMA arises from the aorta 1.5 cm below the celiac trunk. The branches of the SMA include the inferior pancreaticoduodenal artery; the jejunal and ileal branches; and the middle colic, right colic, and ileocolic arteries. The SMA is responsible for the blood supply to the lower part of the pancreas, jejunum, ileum, the ascending colon, and the proximal half of the transverse colon. The IMA originates from the aorta 4 cm above its bifurcation. It gives off the left colic artery and sigmoid branches, and continues as the superior hemorrhoidal artery. It supplies the large bowel from the midtransverse colon to the rectum. The rectum is also supplied by the middle and inferior hemorrhoidal arteries, which arise from the internal iliac artery.

The collateral pathways between the mesenteric arteries are:

- The marginal artery of Drummond, which is derived by the confluence of the right, middle, and left colic arteries, and runs along the mesenteric border of the colon
- The arc of Riolan, which is a branch of the left colic artery communicating with the middle colic artery; is located more centrally in the mesentery; and represents a collateral pathway between the SMA and the IMA
- The hemorrhoidal arteries, which form a collateral system between the IMA and the internal iliac arteries
- The gastroduodenal and pancreaticoduodenal arteries, which form collaterals between celiac trunk and the SMA
- The inferior phrenic arteries, which originate from the abdominal aorta and have posterior branches that anastomose with intercostal arteries, and anterior branches that anastomose with the controlateral artery and with branches of the hepatic artery
- The arc of Buhler, which represents a persistence of the embryonic ventral anastomosis between the SMA and the celiac arterial systems, and which occurs at an unknown rate believed to be 4% or less
- The arc of Barkow, which consists of arteries in the omentum that connect left and right gastroepiploic arteries

The mesenteric venous blood is drained by the portal vein, which is formed by the confluence of splenic vein and superior mesenteric vein (SMV). The mesenteric veins are parallel to the correspondent arteries. The inferior mesenteric vein (IMV) receives supply from the left colic, sigmoid, and superior hemorrhoidal veins. The IMV joins the splenic vein before its confluence with the SMV. The SMV receives the duodenal, pancreatic, right gastroepiploic, jejunal, ileal, right colic, and middle colic veins. The coronary veins (right and left gastric) drain directly into the portal vein.[6,7]

PHYSIOLOGY

The small and large bowels at rest are perfused by 10% to 15% of the cardiac output. After a meal, the splanchnic blood flow can increase to up to 35% of the cardiac output. Seventy percent of this blood flow supplies the mucosa and submucosa. Partly because of increased oxygen extraction, the intestine is able to compensate for an acute reduction in mesenteric blood flow of approximately 75% for up to 12 hours without substantial injury.[8]

Intestinal blood flow is regulated by both intrinsic and extrinsic factors (**Box 1**). Tissue metabolites, such as hydrogen ions (H^+) and potassium ions (K^+), and myogenic mechanisms seem to be involved in the autoregulation of the blood flow. The autoregulation mechanism tries to maintain a constant and adequate blood flow to the bowel despite acute changes in systemic blood pressure. Nitric oxide, produced by endothelial cells, acts as a vasodilator in the regulation of blood flow of the alimentary tract. Prostaglandins are produced in the gastrointestinal tract and include both vasodilators and vasoconstrictors. Prostacyclin (PGI2) and prostaglandin E2 (PGE2) are the main vasodilators. Thromboxane A2 (TxA2) is the major vasoconstrictor. In the resting bowel, the synthesis of vasodilator prostaglandins seems to be predominant as cycloxigenase inhibition reduces intestinal blood flow. Leukotrienes are also derived from arachidonic acid via a different enzymatic

Box 1

Intrinsic and extrinsic mediators in the regulation of gastrointestinal blood flow

Intrinsic

Vasoconstrictors

Leukotrienes

TxA2

Vasodilators

H^+ and K^+

Nitric oxide

PGI2 and PGE2

Extrinsic

Vasoconstrictors

Sympathetic

Angiotensin II

Vasopressin

Somatostatin

Vasodilators

Parasympathetic

Cholecystokinin

Secretin

Enteroglucagonlike peptide

Gastrin

Substance P

Vasoactive intestinal peptide

Gastric inhibitory polypeptide

pathway, lipoxygenase. The cysteinyl leukotrienes (LTC4, LTD4, and LTE4) mediate mesenteric vasoconstriction.[7,9]

The autonomic nervous system is an important extrinsic mechanism of regulation of intestinal perfusion. Parasympathetic fibers cause vasodilation in the stomach and distal colon by increasing endothelial synthesis of nitric oxide. The sympathetic system causes vasoconstriction in the entire alimentary tract via alpha-adrenergic receptors.[10] Angiotensin II and vasopressin are important hormonal vasoconstrictors. Cholecystokinin, secretin, enteroglucagonlike peptide, and gastrin act as vasodilators. Somatostatin causes vasoconstriction in the upper gastrointestinal tract only at pharmacologic doses. Substance P, vasoactive intestinal peptide, and gastric inhibitory polypeptide mediate vasodilation only at pharmacologic doses. Some of these hormones may contribute to the increased intestinal blood flow following a meal.[7,9]

ETIOLOGY

Intestinal ischemia in all its clinical manifestations can be described as an imbalance between oxygen supply and oxygen demand of the intestine. According to the severity and duration of ischemia, lesions may range from patchy mucosal necrosis to transmural necrosis. The mucosa is the layer most susceptible to ischemia. Even a short period of ischemia (eg, 1 hour) may jeopardize intestinal epithemium. Severe and longer ischemia can cause transmural necrosis of the bowel wall with perforation and peritonitis. Chronic ischemia may lead to stricture and bowel obstruction.[11]

The conditions that can cause intestinal ischemia can be grouped into three classes (**Box 2**):

- Presplancnic: all conditions causing a decreased total mesenteric blood flow, hemorrhage, hypovolemia, heart failure
- Splancnic: all conditions that decrease blood flow at local level, like embolus or thrombosis
- Postsplancnic: venous disease

The most common form of presplancnic mesenteric ischemia is NOMI. It is related to decreased

Box 2

Causes of mesenteric ischemia

Presplancnic

Hemorrhage

Hypovolemia

Acute myocardial infarction

Congestive heart failure

Dialysis

Splancnic

Embolism

Thrombosis

Atherosclerosis

Arterial fibrodysplasia

Connective tissue disease

Surgery

Trauma

Compression

Drugs (digitalis, cyclosporine, ergot, pressors)

Postsplancnic

Primary mesenteric venous thrombosis

Hypercoagulable syndromes

Cirrhosis

Abdominal surgery/trauma

cardiac output from decreased preload, contractility, or afterload. Hemorrhagic shock, dehydration, hemodialysis, acute myocardial infarction, and congestive heart failure are common causes of NOMI. NOMI seems to cause 9% of deaths occurring during hemodialysis. The treatment of NOMI is based on resolution of hypotension and administration of papaverine. Papaverine relaxes the vascular smooth muscle by inhibiting the intracellular breakdown of cyclic nucleotides (cyclic adenosine monophosphate, cyclic guanosine monophosphate).[7,9]

PATHOPHYSIOLOGY

During mesenteric ischemia, bowel injury is mediated by two different mechanisms: ischemia and reperfusion.

The reperfusion of ischemic bowel is associated to worsening injury. Parks and Granger[12] found that the histologic changes of the mucosa after 3 hours of ischemia and 1 hour of reperfusion were worse than those associated to 4 hours of ischemia. Experimental studies showed that reperfusion injury is associated with:

- increased microvascular permeability;
- increased epithelial permeability with leaking of fluid and molecules into the bowel lumen; and
- decreased intestinal blood flow.

A study with labeled plasma proteins showed increased vascular permeability to macromolecules after reperfusion.[13] The intestinal epithelial permeability was evaluated by studying the blood-to-lumen movement of 51Cr-labeled EDTA. The intestinal epithelium is usually not very permeable to EDTA. After short ischemia-reperfusion the concentration of EDTA in the bowel lumen was found sevenfold higher than that in controls.[11] Acute occlusion of the SMA is associated with immediate splancnic vasodilatation. If SMA occlusion persists for more than 30 minutes, splancnic vasoconstriction occurs and continues after resolution of SMA occlusion.[9]

After ischemia and reperfusion, the levels of TxA2 and LTC4 in the bowel increase more than 300%. They both have important vasoconstrictor and proinflammatory effects. Prolonged decreased splancnic blood flow (more than 30 minutes) followed by reperfusion is also associated to decreased release of PGI2, a potent vasodilator. Superoxide dismutase, a scavenger of oxygen free radicals, can restore the levels of PGI2 and the SMA blood flow, previously decreased by reperfusion injury. This supports the role of oxygen free radicals as regulators of PGI2 synthesis.[14]

Oxygen-derived free radicals, as superoxide anions, hydrogen peroxide, and hydroxyl radicals, play an important role in the intestinal reperfusion injury. During ischemia, ATP is metabolized to hypoxanthine. After reperfusion, oxygen becomes available to react with hypoxanthine to form xanthine and superoxide anions. Oxygen radicals cause tissue injury directly by peroxidating plasma membrane lipids, breaking DNA strands, and compromising energetic metabolism and calcium exchange. They can antagonize vasodilation mechanisms based on nitric oxide and prostacyclin. Oxygen radicals also trigger local inflammatory response by activating granulocytes and complement.[15]

Neutrophils are important cellular components of reperfusion injury. In experimental studies, depletion of neutrophils or inhibition of neutrophil-endothelial adhesion prevents the effects of reperfusion injury on the ischemic bowel. During reperfusion, neutrophils are activated and infiltrate the bowel wall, contributing to the tissue injury. Activated neutrophils inhibit the release of PGI2 and generate cytotoxic molecules, such as oxygen radicals, proteases, and collagenase. Neutrophil activation is mediated by oxygen radicals, complement anaphylatoxins C3a and C5a, platelet activating factor, leukotriene B4, and TxA2.[16]

Both classical and alternate complement pathways are involved in the reperfusion injury. The soluble complement receptor 1 seems to decrease the histologic alterations related to the reperfusion injury. Complement contributes to the tissue damage by forming the membrane attack complex and activating local inflammation.[17]

Nitric oxide is released constitutively by endothelium and protects the mucosa from damage due to reperfusion injury. Inhibition of the endothelial nitric oxide–synthase is associated with vasoconstriction, a threefold increase in protein extravasation, a twofold increase in mucosal permeability, and a 15-fold increase in neutrophil adhesion to postcapillary venules.[11,13] Nitric oxide activates a pathway involving cyclic guanosine monophosphate, platelet-activating factor, and endothelial cytoskeleton responsible for the regulation of microvascular permeability to proteins.[18]

During reperfusion, eicosanoids, complement, endotoxin, and cytokines are released into the circulation. They mediate systemic effects, including systemic inflammatory response syndrome and injury to the lungs (adult respiratory distress syndrome), liver, heart, and kidney, which can complicate intestinal ischemia.[19] The lung injury is characterized by increased microvascular permeability and pulmonary vasoconstriction. Neutrophils are the main cellular component in the pathogenesis of this injury. The liver involvement in the reperfusion injury is consistent with oxidant stress: Release of hepatocellular enzymes, reduced liver perfusion, and bile synthesis are the main effects of this injury. Decreased cardiac contraction-relaxation function and reduced renal blood flow are other important systemic components of reperfusion injury. In many of these responses, eicosanoids, especially TxA2, seem to play the role of main molecular mediators.[9] The poor prognosis of severe acute mesenteric ischemia seems to be related to the development of a multiple organ failure syndrome.[20]

ACUTE MESENTERIC ISCHEMIA

Acute mesenteric ischemia is a potentially life-threatening condition. Its mortality ranges from 30% to 65%. The majority of patients are over the age 60. Abdominal pain is the most common presenting symptom (94%). Patients usually complain of abdominal pain out of proportion to the abdominal examination. Other symptoms include nausea (56%), vomiting (38%), diarrhea (31%), and tachycardia (31%). A patient's temperature may be normal in the early course. Fever may indicate bowel necrosis. Melena or occult blood may occur in up to 75% of patients. On physical examination, the abdomen is usually soft and minimally tender at the onset of acute ischemia. Peritoneal signs with tenderness and guarding will develop in case of bowel infarction.[21]

In patients with acute mesenteric ischemia, it is important to differentiate between occlusive causes (embolism, thrombosis) and nonocclusive causes (NOMI). Acute mesenteric ischemia due to arterial occlusion needs an operative treatment while NOMI can be treated nonoperatively unless there is evidence of gangrenous bowel.

The most common causes of acute mesenteric ischemia are:

- Embolization: 50%
- Arterial thrombosis: 25%
- NOMI: 20%
- Venous thrombosis: 5%[22]

The most frequent cause of acute mesenteric ischemia is an embolus to the SMA. The sources of emboli may include the left atrium (most common) in patients with atrial fibrillation, the left ventricle in cases of ventricular mural thrombus, and aortic aneurysm. These patients usually do not have a previous history of chronic mesenteric ischemia. Their past medical history is usually remarkable for atrial fibrillation (up to 70%), myocardial infarction, rheumatic heart disease, and arterial emboli. In most cases, patients with chronic atrial fibrillation were on adequate anticoagulation when they developed acute mesenteric ischemia. Because the embolic arterial occlusion is an acute event, the collateral circulation is usually limited. The severity of embolic disease and the delay in diagnosis may explain the high mortality rate (70%).[23] Most of the emboli affect the SMA because of the acute angle of origin of the SMA from the aorta. Emboli to the SMA usually stop beyond the takeoff of the middle colic artery. Because this location is distal to the origin of the inferior pancreaticoduodenal artery, there is less chance for collateral flow. Emboli may also distribute to branches of the SMA: the middle colic artery (55%), the right colic artery (16%), the ileocolic artery (7%), and the small peripheral branches (4%). The celiac trunk is less frequently affected by symptomatic emboli because of its right angle of takeoff from the aorta. An embolus in the celiac trunk usually lodges at the trifurcation, allowing enough collateral flow from the SMA. Emboli to the IMA are rare and may occur after manipulation of an atherosclerotic aorta. The most common presentation is infarction of the sigmoid colon.[7]

Thrombosis usually is the complication of atherosclerosis in the mesenteric vessels. The common site of atherosclerotic plaque and thrombosis is at the origin of the mesenteric vessels. The SMA is the most common affected artery, followed by the celiac trunk and the IMA. At least 50% of these patients have a previous history of abdominal pain, weight loss, and diarrhea. Their medical history is usually remarkable for other localizations of atherosclerosis, such as coronary artery disease, cerebrovascular disease, and peripheral vascular disease. The risk factors for SMA thrombosis are the same as those for atherosclerosis and include advanced age, smoking, hyperlipidemia, diabetes, and sedentary lifestyle.

Leukocytosis, elevated lactate and amylase, and high anion gap metabolic acidosis are the most common but not specific laboratory findings in acute mesenteric ischemia. CT scan accuracy in diagnosing acute mesenteric ischemia is reported as 58%.[21] CT angiography showed a 94% positive predictive value in animal studies. Angiography is the gold standard in diagnosis of acute mesenteric ischemia because (1) it localizes the site of occlusion to better plan the revascularization; and (2) it enables balloon angioplasty and stenting to be used for revascularization, especially in patients with high operative risk without frank peritoneal signs.

The benefit of early angiography was demonstrated in a series in which a 67% survival rate was observed in patients with acute SMA embolism when a protocol involving prompt angiography was initiated within 12 hours of the suspected event. This is a vast improvement from the 70% mortality rate observed in the late 1960s.[4]

Fogarty catheter embolectomy can be used in patients with embolic mesenteric occlusion. Because of the risk of thrombosis at the site of arteriotomy (17%), the arterial closure is performed with a patch angioplasty.[24] Mesenteric bypass is performed in case of thrombotic occlusion. In anterograde mesenteric bypass, the donor vessel is the supraceliac aorta, while in the retrograde bypass, the inflow source is the infrarenal aorta or the iliac artery. Anterograde bypass is more challenging, but involves the supraceliac aorta, which is usually less affected by atherosclerotic disease. Revascularization to at least two mesenteric arteries is performed to restore a complete blood supply and to prevent future ischemic episodes. The 5-year patency rate of aortomesenteric bypass is 89% to 94%. Bowel resection is necessary in case of bowel necrosis (30% of cases). A second-look operation is considered when "questionable" but not frankly necrotic bowel loops are left in the first procedure.[7]

NOMI can be defined as mesenteric ischemia in the presence of patent mesenteric vessels. Risk factors for NOMI include congestive heart failure, cardiac arrhythmias, cardiac bypass, hemodialysis, shock, medications (digitalis, cyclosporine, ergot alkaloids, vasopressors), and drugs (cocaine). All the conditions with low cardiac output predispose to mesenteric ischemia. Mesenteric vasoconstriction occurs and is activated by both angiotensin and vasopressin. If this vasoconstriction persists for more than 30 minutes, it becomes irreversible. Delayed correction of low cardiac output is associated with persistence of mesenteric vasoconstriction. Mesenteric ischemia has been associated with bacterial translocation. Thirteen of 33 patients who had a cardiac arrest (average duration 13 minutes) became bacteremic with enteric bacteria within 12 hours.[25] Chronic hemodialysis patients with NOMI should be treated with immediate reversal of hypotension and papaverin infusion.[26] NOMI has been described after starting enteral feeding without any other apparent cause. Feeding increases the intestinal demand for blood supply and can cause demand ischemia in patients with borderline blood supply. Some medications, such as digitalis and cyclosporine, cause vasoconstriction with a calcium-dependent mechanism. Calcium channel blockers are able to reverse this pharmacologic-induced splancnic vasoconstriction.[27] The ischemic injury associated with NOMI usually localizes in the small bowel. Right colon ischemia has been described as nonocclusive ischemia in trauma patients in hemorrhagic shock.[28] The initial treatment of NOMI is intra-arterial infusion of vasodilators (papaverine, glucagone, prostaglandins) with concomitant intravenous fluid resuscitation. In the absence of peritoneal signs, a conservative management is warranted.

CHRONIC MESENTERIC ISCHEMIA

Chronic mesenteric ischemia (also called intestinal angina) refers to chronic episodic or continuous intestinal hypoperfusion, which usually develops in patients with mesenteric atherosclerotic disease. Patients are usually elderly, heavy smokers, and have diffuse atherosclerotic disease. They complain of chronic postprandial pain, weight loss, and diarrhea, and often have arterial occlusive lesions in the splancnic arteries. Abdominal pain, usually dull and crampy, begins within 30 minutes after eating and lasts 1 to 3 hours.

Because of the extensive collateral flow, at least two of the three splancnic arteries usually need to be occluded to cause clinically relevant symptoms. Isolated stenotic lesions of the SMA distal to the middle colic branch can also produce chronic ischemia by excluding any collateral flow.[29] Causes of chronic mesenteric ischemia include atherosclerosis (most common), arterial fibrodysplasia, and connective tissue disease.

The clinical manifestations of chronic mesenteric ischemia are related to the rapidity of progression of the arterial narrowing and to the development of collaterals. The finding of a stenosis in splancnic arteries alone is not diagnostic for chronic mesenteric ischemia. Up to 18% of individuals over 65 in the general population have significant stenosis of the celiac artery or SMA without symptoms.[30]

Duplex scan is a good screening test to detect occlusion at the origin of the celiac and mesenteric arteries. Magnetic resonance angiography and CT angiography correlate very well with conventional angiography and are reproducible from observer to observer. The treatment of chronic mesenteric ischemia includes both percutaneous endovascular procedures and open surgical procedures. Primary graft patency rates after surgical revascularization range from 57% to 69% at 5 years. The freedom-from-recurrence rates at 5 years and 10 years are approximately 80% and 60%, respectively.[31] Percutaneous transluminal angioplasty was initially introduced as an alternative to surgery for patients with chronic mesenteric ischemia who were poor surgical candidates. Most studies report success rates of greater than 80%.[32] Resolution of abdominal pain has been achieved in 75% to 100% of patients and half of the patients experienced weight gain. Eighty percent of patients were free of symptoms at 2 to 3 years. Recurrent symptoms are usually associated with restenosis, which can often be successfully managed with repeat angioplasty.[33]

MESENTERIC VENOUS THROMBOSIS

Mesenteric venous thrombosis (MVT) is responsible for 5% to 15% of bowel ischemia. It is more common in the fifth and sixth decades of life. MVT includes acute, subacute, and chronic forms. Acute MVT occurs when the major mesenteric veins are occluded. Patients present with severe abdominal pain, distention, and positive fecal occult blood. Subacute MVT is usually caused by thrombosis of smaller mesenteric veins. This form has a slow insidious onset and evolves over days with vague abdominal pain and nausea. Chronic MVT lasts several weeks or months.

MVT is defined as primary in cases where no apparent cause of mesenteric venous occlusion is evident. Secondary MVT includes all mesenteric venous occlusions with known predisposing conditions. In 60% to 80% of MVT, a predisposing cause was identified. The causes of MVT include hypercoagulable states, venous stasis, and inflammation. The available data suggest that the most common disorder is the factor V Leiden mutation (causing resistance to activated protein C), which is present in 20% to 40% of patients.[34] Other hypercoagulable states include such hematologic conditions as antithrombin III deficiency, protein C and S deficiency, polycythemia vera, thrombocytosis, hyperfibrinogenemia, and myeloproliferative disorders. Hypercoagulability is also associated with use of oral contraceptives and neoplasms of the gastrointestinal tract, pancreas, lung, and ovary. Patients after surgery are at increased risk for MVT. Splenectomy is the procedure with the highest risk for MVT. Most MVTs occur within 1 month after splenectomy. Abdominal trauma, abdominal inflammation, peritonitis, and portal hypertension are other risk factors for MVT.

Acute MVT has high incidence of recurrence (33%–40%) in the early postoperative period, so that many clinicians perform a second-look operation either routinely or selectively. In the case of selective second-look operations, the choice to perform a second-look procedure is based on the lack of clear demarcation zones at the first operation, leaving questionable zones of intestine not resected and left for observation.[35]

MVT without peritoneal signs can be managed conservatively. Early systemic anticoagulation with heparin is the main nonoperative treatment and improves survival.[1,36] In a study of 72 patients with MVT, 64% underwent exploratory laparotomy, of whom 85% had bowel necrosis requiring resection.[35]

ISCHEMIC COLITIS

Ischemic colitis, the most common form of intestinal ischemia, represents 50% to 60% of all cases of gastrointestinal ischemia. Ischemic colitis can be gangrenous or nongangrenous. The nongangrenous forms account for 80% to 85% of the cases and include transient and chronic forms.[37,38] In the nongangrenous transient type, there is edema, hemorrhage, and possible necrosis of the mucosa and submucosa. This form usually resolves with a complete anatomic and functional recovery in 2 weeks. The nongangrenous chronic form usually extends to the muscularis propria. The damaged muscularis is usually replaced by fibrous tissue, resulting in colonic strictures. Gangrenous forms comprise the 15% to 20% of cases of ischemic colitis and are characterized by transmural necrosis, evolving in sepsis and usually requiring surgical resection.

An acute decrease in the colonic blood supply is usually the cause of ischemic colitis. In most cases of ischemic colitis, the cause is not apparent (idiopathic). Known causes of ischemic colitis include:

- Mesenteric vascular occlusion
- Shock
- Medications (digitalis, catecholamines, estrogen, danazol, gold, nonsteroidal anti-inflammatory medications, neuroleptics, diuretics and laxatives)
- Cocaine
- Colonic obstruction
- Infection with *Escherichia coli*

Vascular occlusion may be related to thrombosis, embolization, trauma, radiologic procedures, or surgical procedures. Small vessel disease may be caused by diabetes mellitus, rheumatoid arthritis, or vasculitis.

Colon ischemia is described as a complication of abdominal aortic surgery in 0.2% to 10% of cases. It is five times more frequent after abdominal aortic aneurysm repair than after revascularization for aortic occlusive disease. In patients with aortic occlusive disease, the IMA is usually occluded and an adequate collateral circulation to the left colon is already established before surgery. In patients with an abdominal aortic aneurysm, intraoperative ligation of IMA can cause ischemia of the left colon in case of inadequate collateral flow. Risk factors for colon ischemia after abdominal aortic aneurysm repair include prolonged cross clamp time, reoperative procedures, ruptured aneurysms, hypoxemia, and hypotension.[39]

Colon involvement is usually segmental. Every part of the colon can be affected. The splenic flexure and the sigmoid colon are the most commonly involved areas. Because of the vascular anatomy of the colon, two places are at particular at risk for ischemia: Griffith's point in the splenic flexure and Sudek's point in the sigmoid. The sigmoid colon is involved in 75% of cases, the splenic flexure in 25%, and the right colon in 10%. A predisposing factor to colon ischemia is the absence of a marginal artery of Drummond at the splenic flexure. This artery is absent in 7% of the population. Ischemic colitis due to low flow states usually affects the right colon in its retroperitoneal surface.

Patients with ischemic colitis are usually elderly and complain of acute abdominal pain, diarrhea, and hematochezia. The blood loss is usually small. The physical examination is remarkable for mild abdominal distention and localized tenderness. The definitive diagnosis of ischemic colitis is based on colonoscopy.

OTHER MESENTERIC ISCHEMIC SYNDROMES

The celiac artery compression syndrome includes all cases of external compression of celiac artery due to the median arcuate ligament or celiac ganglia. Patients usually complain of postprandial abdominal pain, positional abdominal pain, nausea, and weight loss.

Mesenteric vessels may be involved in vasculitis with consequent bowel ischemia. Vasculitis may affect the main arteries (eg, Takayasu arteritis, giant cell arteritis), medium-sized arteries (eg, polyarteritis nodosa, Buerger's disease, Kawasaki disease), or the small vessels (eg, Henoch-Schonlein syndrome, systemic lupus erythematosus, rheumatoid arthritis, Wegener granulomatosis).[40]

Cocaine abuse is associated with both acute and chronic ischemia. Chronic ischemia may be due to thrombotic occlusion of both the celiac artery and the SMA.[40]

SUMMARY

Mesenteric ischemia includes several clinical syndromes caused by inadequate blood flow to the intestine. The causes of these disorders can be classified as presplancnic (eg, NOMI), splancnic (eg, embolism, thrombosis, atherosclerosis), and postsplancnic (eg, MVT). The mechanisms of ischemic bowel injury are related to both ischemia and reperfusion. Oxygen-derived free radicals contribute to the reperfusion injury by directly causing tissue injury, altering eicosanoid metabolism, and activating neutrophils and complement. Understanding the etiology and pathogenesis of the different intestinal ischemic syndromes is necessary for an adequate clinical management of these disorders. Acute mesenteric ischemia is caused by embolic or thrombotic mesenteric occlusion, states of low blood perfusion and vasospasm without vessel occlusion, and MVT. In most cases, chronic mesenteric ischemia is caused by atherosclerotic stenosis of mesenteric vessels. Ischemic colitis can be caused by either mesenteric occlusion or hypoperfusion states. Early diagnosis and treatment are the keys to improved results in the management of mesenteric ischemia. Despite the advances of diagnostic techniques, a high index of clinical suspicion seems necessary for the early detection and treatment of these disorders.

REFERENCES

1. Herbert GS, Steele SR. Acute and chronic mesenteric ischemia. Surg Clin North Am 2007;87: 1115–34.
2. Martinez JP, Hogan GJ. Mesenteric ischemia. Emerg Med Clin North Am 2004;22(4):909–28.
3. Acosta S, Ogren M, Sternby NH, et al. Incidence of acute thrombo-embolic occlusion of the superior mesenteric artery—a population-based study. Eur J Vasc Endovasc Surg 2004;27(2):145–50.
4. Boley SJ, Brandt LJ, Sammartano RJ. History of mesenteric ischemia. The evolution of a diagnosis and management. Surg Clin North Am 1997;77: 275–88.
5. Boley SJ, Sammartano RJ, Brandt LJ. Historical perspective. In: Longo WE, Peterson GJ, Jacobs DJ, editors. Intestinal ischemia disorders. St. Louis (MO): Quality Medical Publishing; 1999. p. 1–15.
6. Hagspiel KD, Angle JF, Spinosa DJ, et al. Angiography: diagnosis and therapeutics. In: Longo WE, Peterson GJ, Jacobs DJ, editors. Intestinal ischemia disorders. St. Louis (MO): Quality Medical Publishing; 1999. p. 105–54.
7. Myers SI, Lowry PA. Circulation and vascular disorders of the splancnic vascular bed. In: Miller TA, editor. Modern surgical care. New York: Informa Healthcare; 2006. p. 381–413.
8. Boley SJ, Frieber W, Winslow PR, et al. Circulatory responses to acute reduction of superior mesenteric arterial flow. Physiologist 1969;12:180.
9. Turnage RH, Myers SI. Pathophysiology. In: Longo WE, Peterson GJ, Jacobs DJ, editors. Intestinal ischemia disorders. St. Louis (MO): Quality Medical Publishing; 1999. p. 1–15.
10. Guyton AC, Hall JE. Nervous regulation of the circulation and rapid control of arterial pressure.

In: Guyton AC, editor. Textbook of medical physiology. Philadelphia: WB Saunders; 2000. p. 184–94.

11. Payne D, Kubes P. Nitric oxide donors reduce the rise in reperfusion-induced intestinal mucosal permeability. Am J Physiol 1993;265:G189–95.

12. Parks DA, Granger DN. Contributions of ischemia and reperfusion to mucosal lesion formation. Am J Physiol 1982;250:G749–53.

13. Kubes P. Ischemia-reperfusion in feline small intestine: a role for nitric oxide. Am J Physiol 1993;264: G143–9.

14. Myers SI, Hernandez R. Oxygen free radical regulation of rat splancnic blood flow. Surgery 1992;112:347–54.

15. Zimmerman BJ, Grisham MB, Granger DN. Mechanism of oxidant-mediated microvascular injury following reperfusion of the ischemic intestine. Basic Life Sci 1986;49:881–6.

16. Kurtel H, Fujimoto K, Zimmerman BJ, et al. Ischemia-reperfusion–induced mucosal dysfunction: role of neutrophils. Am J Physiol 1991;261:G490–6.

17. Hill J, Lindsay TF, Ortiz F, et al. Soluble complement receptor 1 ameliorates the local and remote organ injury after intestinal ischemia-reperfusion in the rat. J Immunol 1992;149:1723–8.

18. Kurose I, Kubes P, Wolf R, et al. Inhibition of nitric oxide production: mechanism of vascular albumin leakage. Circ Res 1993;73:164–72.

19. Oldham KT, Guice KS, Turnage RH, et al. The systemic consequences of intestinal ischemia/reperfusion injury. J Vasc Surg 1993;93:136–7.

20. Yasuhara H. Acute mesenteric ischemia: the challenge of gastroenterology. Surg Today 2005;35(3):185–95.

21. Kougias P, Lau D, El Sayed H, et al. Determinants of mortality and treatment outcome following surgical interventions for acute mesenteric ischemia. J Vasc Surg 2007;46:467–74.

22. Stoney R, Cunningham C. Acute mesenteric ischemia. Surgery 1993;114:489–90.

23. Schoots IG, Koffeman GI, Legemate DA, et al. Systematic review of survival after acute mesenteric ischemia according to the disease etiology. Br J Surg 2004;91:17–27.

24. Levi PJ, Krausz MM, Manny J. The role of second-look procedure in improving survival time for patients with mesenteric venous thrombosis. Surg Gynecol Obstet 1990;170:287–91.

25. Gaussorgues P, Gueugniaud PY, Vedrinne JM, et al. Bacteremia following cardiac arrest and cardiopulmonary resuscitation. Intensive Care Med 1988;4:575–7.

26. Diamond SM, Emmett M, Henrich WL. Bowel infarction as a cause of death in dialysis patients. JAMA 1986;256:2545–7.

27. Rego A, Vargas R, Suarez KR, et al. Mechanism of cyclosporine potentiation of vasoconstriction of the isolated rat mesenteric arterial bed: role of extracellular calcium. J Pharmacol Exp Ther 1990;254: 799–808.

28. Ludwig KA, Quebbeman EJ, Bergstein JM, et al. Shock-associated right colon ischemia and necrosis. J Trauma 1995;39:1171–4.

29. Levy AD. Mesenteric ischemia. Radiol Clin North Am 2007;45:593–9.

30. Wilson DB, Mostafavi K, Craven TE, et al. Clinical course of mesenteric artery stenosis in elderly Americans. Arch Intern Med 2006;166:2095–100.

31. Cho JS, Carr JA, Jacobsen G, et al. Long-term outcome after mesenteric artery reconstruction: a 37-year experience. J Vasc Surg 2002;35:453–60.

32. Allen RC, Martin GH, Rees CR, et al. Mesenteric angioplasty in the treatment of chronic intestinal ischemia. J Vasc Surg 1996;24:415–21.

33. Matsumoto AH, Angle JF, Spinosa DJ, et al. Percutaneous transluminal angioplasty and stenting in the treatment of chronic mesenteric ischemia: results and longterm followup. J Am Coll Surg 2002;194: S22–31.

34. Thomas DP, Roberts HR. Hypercoagulability in venous and arterial thrombosis. Ann Intern Med 1997;126:638–44.

35. Rhee RY, Gloviczki P, Mendonca CT, et al. Mesenteric venous thrombosis: still a lethal disease in the 1990s. J Vasc Surg 1994;20:688–97.

36. Rhee RY, Gloviczki P. Mesenteric venous thrombosis. Surg Clin North Am 1997;77:327–38.

37. Brandt LJ, Boley SJ. Colonic ischemia. Surg Clin North Am 1992;72:203–29.

38. Fitzgerald SF, Kaminiski DL. Ischemic colitis. Semin Colon Rectal Surg 1993;4:222–8.

39. Brewster DC, Franklin DP, Cambria RP, et al. Intestinal ischemia complicating abdominal aortic surgery. Surgery 1991;109:447–54.

40. Myers SI, Clagett GP, Valentine ME, et al. Chronic intestinal ischemia caused by intravenous cocaine use: report of two cases and review of the literature. J Vasc Surg 1996;23:724–9.

Clinical Symptoms of Intestinal Vascular Disorders

Giovanni Bartone, MD[a],*, Beatrice Ulloa Severino, MD[a],
Mariano Fortunato Armellino, MD[b],
Mauro Natale Domenico Maglio, MD[a], Maurizio Castriconi, MD[a]

KEYWORDS

- Intestinal ischemia • Acute mesenteric ischemia
- Mesenteric vein thrombosis
- Nonocclusive mesenteric ischemia
- Chronic mesenteric ischemia • Symptoms

The pathogenesis and symptoms of intestinal ischemia are extremely variable and complex and, despite scientific advances, intestinal ischemia still represents a challenge for the surgeon because of the high mortality rate.

The onset of the illness is related to the cause of intestinal ischemia, which can be classified into thrombotic or nonthrombotic ischemia. The thrombotic events include the occlusion of the superior mesenteric artery (SMA) because of a thrombosis or an embolism, or a thrombosis of the superior mesenteric vein (**Table 1**).[1]

Obviously, patients with an arterial intestinal ischemia usually present with either a cardiac arrhythmia with an underlying atherosclerosis.[2] The nonocclusive mesenteric ischemia (NOMI) is the consequence of a splanchnic hypoperfusion, which may be related to local or general causes. Among the local causes are a strangulated hernia, intussusception, a volvulus, or adhesive bands that determine a bowel obstruction with hypoperfusion. The general causes determining a NOMI are all the situations with a secondary vasoconstriction from a severe hypovolemia, following a cardiac failure, inflammation, or septic shock.

Regardless of the events determining a mesenteric ischemia, the final result is a broad spectrum of bowel damage, ranging from minimal and reversible alterations to a complete hemorrhagic necrosis of the intestinal wall.

The symptoms of acute mesenteric ischemia (AMI) can appear quite suddenly in a patient with an apparently good state of health, and although it is rare, it has had an increasing incidence parallel to the aging population in recent decades.[3] In spite of a prompt diagnosis and an aggressive therapy, the mesenteric ischemia still has a high rate of mortality, ranging from 60% to 90%, related to how quickly therapeutic measures are taken.[1,4–6]

The first symptoms of an acute arterial mesenteric ischemia, especially in the case of an embolic origin and less if thrombotic, are absolutely aspecific with a sudden onset and a rapid worsening of the clinical condition of the patient. Instead, in mesenteric venous ischemia and in NOMI there is a gradual onset of symptoms and a more protracted clinical course.[7]

The patient with an embolic AMI complains of a sudden and persistent abdominal pain in the periumbilical area and in the left abdominal quadrant, with a discrepancy between a severe abdominal pain and minimal clinical findings. The clinical findings of a peritonitis, such as a muscular defense or Blumberg's sign, are not evident from touching the abdomen in an early phase.[8] The abdominal pain is followed by or associated with

a Department of General and Emergency Surgery, "A. Cardarelli" Hospital, Naples, Italy
b Department of General and Emergency Surgery with Polyspecialistic Observation, "A. Cardarelli" Hospital, Naples, Italy
* Corresponding author. Via Scipione Capece 2/c, 80122 Naples, Italy.
E-mail address: giovanni.bartone@ospedalecardarelli.it (G. Bartone).

Radiol Clin N Am 46 (2008) 887–889
doi:10.1016/j.rcl.2008.08.005
0033-8389/08/$ – see front matter © 2008 published by Elsevier Inc.

Table 1
Clinical symptoms related to risk factors of mesenteric ischemia

Cause	Risk Factors	Presentation
Arterial embolism	Arrhythmia Myocardial infarction Rheumatic valve disease, endocarditis Cardiomyopathy Ventricular aneurysms History of embolic events Recent angiography	Sudden onset of abdominal pain Nausea Vomiting Hematochezia Melena Hypotension Peritonitis

Arterial thrombosis	Atherosclerosis
	Prolonged hypotension
	Estrogen
	Hypercoagulability
		Insidious onset with
		  progression to
		  constant pain

Nonocclusive	Hypovolemia Hypotension Low cardiac output status α-adrenergic agonists Digoxin β-receptor blocking agents	Acute or subacute Abdominal distension and tenderness Muscular defense Hypotension Fever Decreased bowel sounds Nausea Sickness Anorexia

Venus thrombosis	Right-sided heart failure
	Previous deep vein thrombosis,
	  hepatosplenomegaly
	Primary clotting disorder,
	  malignancy
	Hepatitis
	Pancreatitis
	Recent abdominal surgery
	  recent abdominal infection
	Estrogens
	Polycythemia
	Sickle cell disease
		Insidious onset of
		  abdominal pain
		Distension and
		  tenderness
		Nausea
		Anorexia
		Fever

nausea, vomiting, and hematochezia,[2] while the signs of a peritonitis and hypotension appear more rarely and at a later stage.[9,10] The latter is related to dehydration because of an excessive fluid loss from the third spacing of fluid, which leads to mental confusion, tachycardia, and tachypnea up to circulatory collapse,[7] with every sign of a septic shock. Only 15% of the cases present melena or hematochezia, but an occult blood test is positive in the stools of nearly 50% of cases.[8] If a large segment of the bowel is ischemic, there are no peristaltic sounds with abdominal auscultation.

Patients with a chronic mesenteric thrombosis frequently report warning signs, such as postprandial abdominal pain and nausea with subsequent weight loss. This slow clinical evolution with a subacute onset leads to the previously described typical AMI.

The difference in onset between the embolic form and thrombotic form of ischemia is related to the poorly developed collateral circulation of the superior mesenteric artery when a sudden event, such as an embolism, takes place. There is a valid possibility of a bowel infarction in a patient with a severe abdominal pain that is out of proportion with that suggested by physical examination, particularly when the patient, over 60 years old, has a history of recent myocardial infarction, congestive heart failure, atrial fibrillation, or arterial emboli.[7]

Even laboratory findings are not sufficient for the diagnosis of bowel ischemia. The main laboratory abnormalities are hemoconcentration, leukocytosis, metabolic acidosis with high anion gap, and lactate concentrations.[7] Some investigators describe an early high level of C-reactive protein.[2]

Other early, but aspecific laboratory abnormalities are high levels of serum amylase, aspartate amino-transferase, lactate dehydrogenase, and creatine phosphokinase, while an hyperphosphatemia and hyperkaliemia are present at later stages and are associated with an irreversible intestinal wall ischemic damage.[7]

The risk factors in mesenteric venous thrombosis (MVT) are prothrombotic states because of heritable or acquired disorders of coagulation, inflammatory bowel diseases, and cancer. Except in the rare fulminating onset, patients with MVT usually come under clinical observation later, usually 1 or 2 weeks after the onset of the symptoms, complaining of diffuse or localized nonspecific abdominal pain associated with anorexia and diarrhea, sometimes with fever and abdominal distension.

Routine blood tests, like those in arterial mesenteric ischemia, are not helpful in the early stage of MVT. Abdominal films are abnormal in 50% to 75% of the patients; a semiopaque indentation of the bowel lumen is an expression of either mucosal edema (thumbprinting) and pneumatosis intestinalis, or free peritoneal air or air in the portal vein is typical of a bowel infarction.[11]

NOMI accounts for 20% to 30% of all causes of AMI, with a mortality rate around 50%. Nonocclusive forms are associated with a low cardiac output, leading to splanchnic hypoperfusion in patients over 50 years of age suffering from myocardial infarction, congestive heart failure, aortic insufficiency, or renal or hepatic disease.[12]

Early symptoms are frequently absent and the typical acute abdominal pain may be the only early symptom of NOMI. An increased blood analysis activity could be found as early as 90 minutes after the onset of ischemia, but are nonspecific. Plain film radiographs of the abdomen show signs of mesenteric ischemia up to 12 to 24 hours after the onset of symptoms. Mesenteric angiography is the only sure test for the diagnosis of suspected AMI. Prognosis is not favorable, with a high mortality rate, related to the delay of diagnosis in a patient in an already bad state of health.

Chronic mesenteric ischemia presents a diffuse postprandial pain (intestinal angina) lasting from 1 to 3 hours and increasing in the long run. This pain results in a sitophobia, the patient, usually an old patient with a severe atherosclerotic stenosis of the SMA, refrains from eating to avoid pain, which causes deterioration in his health.[13]

The result of any form of mesenteric ischemia, acute or chronic, occlusive or nonocclusive, is bowel infarction. When it occurs, clinical signs of peritonitis, hemodynamic instability, sepsis, and multiorgan failure will be evident.

SUMMARY

Despite advances made in the diagnostic and therapeutic field, acute intestinal ischemia remains a highly lethal condition. This is related to the variability of symptoms and the absence of typical laboratory alterations in early stage. In fact, the clinical onset of acute mesenteric ischemia is aspecific, characterized by a sudden and diffuse abdominal pain and the signs and symptoms of an acute abdomen appear only with bowel infarction.

REFERENCES

1. Martinez JP, Hogan GJ. Mesenteric ischemia. Emerg Med Clin North Am 2004;22:909–28.
2. Kassahun WT, Schulz T, Richter O, et al. Unchanged high mortality rates from acute occlusive intestinal ischemia: six year review. Langenbecks Arch Surg 2008;393(2):163–71.
3. Stoney RJ, Cunningham CG. Acute mesenteric ischemia. Surgery 1993;114:489–90.
4. Brandt LJ, Boley SJ. AGA technical review on intestinal ischemia. Gastroenterology 2000;118:954–68.
5. Sachs SM, Morton JH, Schwartz SI. Acute mesenteric ischemia. Surgery 1982;92:646–53.
6. Klempnauer J, Grothues F, Bektas H, et al. Longterm results after surgery for acute mesenteric ischemia. Surgery 1997;121:239–43.
7. Oldenburg WA, Lau LL, Rodenberg TJ, et al. Acute mesenteric ischemia: a clinical review. Arch Intern Med 2004;164(10):1054–62.
8. Sreenarasimhaiah J. Diagnosis and management of intestinal ischaemic disorders. BMJ 2003;326(7403): 1372–6.
9. Edwards MS, Cherr GS, Craven TE, et al. Acute occlusive mesenteric ischemia: surgical management and outcomes. Ann Vasc Surg 2003;17(1):72–9.
10. Grendell JH, Ockner RK. Mesenteric venous thrombosis. Gastroenterology 1982;82:358–72.
11. Kumar S, Sarr MG, Kamath PS. Mesenteric venous thrombosis. N Engl J Med 2001;345(23):1683–8.
12. Trompeter M, Brazda T, Remy CT, et al. Nonocclusive mesenteric ischemia: etiology, diagnosis, and interventional therapy. Eur Radiol 2002;12(5): 1179–87.
13. Sreenarasimhaiah J. Diagnosis and management of ischemic colitis. Curr Gastroenterol Rep 2005;7(5): 421–6.

Small Bowel Vascular Disorders from Arterial Etiology and Impaired Venous Drainage

Stefania Romano, MD[a],*, Raffaella Niola, MD[b],
Franco Maglione, MD[b], Luigia Romano, MD[a]

KEYWORDS

- Small bowel ischemia • Infarction • MDCT
- Acute abdomen

Vascular disorders of the intestine represent a common pathologic entity to diagnose in emergency situations. Sensibility and specificity of the imaging findings are not easy to recognize and interpret without knowledge on how the small intestine reacts to the arterial or venous flow alterations and what the consequent modification is in its morphology, dynamism, and imaging appearance. The search for the "best" imaging method could be unnecessary in the absence of a well-defined "scheme" of possible manifestations or spectrum of findings of the disease. Because the clinical entity of ischemia of the intestine is the result of an imbalance between nutrient and oxygen demand and available oxygen, clinical problems that have an adverse effect of the intestinal oxygen supply can cause impaired intestinal viability and function.[1] Of the blood flow devoted to the intestine at rest, 70% to 90% supplies the mucosal-submucosal layers; the remainder supplies the muscularis.[1] Intestinal perfusion is presumed to be regulated by intrinsic, extrinsic, and circulating determinants.[1] Acute intestinal ischemia reperfusion damage can be caused by three main categories of conditions:[1] (1) presplanchnic (any clinical pathology that implies a decreased splanchnic blood flow by reduced cardiac output or "nonocclusive ischemia");[1] (2) splanchnic (any pathologic event that causes decreased blood flow at the level of the splanchnic bed, such as arterial embolus and thrombosis);[1] (3) postsplanchnic (any condition that leads to a decrease in splanchnic blood flow with an increase in venous pressure and resultant reflex splanchnic arterial vasoconstriction, such as mesenteric venous thrombosis).[1]

Injury to the intestine causes an appearance of the wall different from the "normal" or basic feature. Because the mucosa and the submucosa layers are much more involved in an ischemic event and manifest different findings depending on the duration and severity of the injury, from a diagnostic radiology point of view, the imaging method that allows investigation of the intestinal wall and abdominal vascular pattern is preferred in the assessment of suspected intestinal ischemia. It is always important to distinguish between ischemia, which can be a reversible event (although damages from reperfusion could be present), and infarction, which is a severe condition characterized by transmural necrosis and may be associated with perforation and peritonitis or multiple organ failure syndrome.[1]

In the emergency evaluation of patients with acute abdominal pain and clinical suspicion of small bowel intestinal ischemia or infarction, time is an essential factor because it represents the critical crossroad between immediate surgery, clinical

[a] Department of Diagnostic Imaging, Section of General and Emergency Radiology, "A. Cardarelli" Hospital, Naples, NA, Italy
[b] Department of Diagnostic Imaging, Section of Vascular and Interventional Radiology, "A. Cardarelli" Hospital, Naples, NA, Italy
* Corresponding author. Via Giuseppe Fava 28 parco la piramide, 80016 Marano di Napoli (NA), Italy.
E-mail address: stefromano@libero.it (S. Romano).

Radiol Clin N Am 46 (2008) 891–908
doi:10.1016/j.rcl.2008.07.003
0033-8389/08/$ – see front matter © 2008 Elsevier Inc. All rights reserved.

observation, and vascular interventional procedures required. The basic imaging methodologies, such as abdominal radiograph and ultrasound, usually are performed during the first-look evaluation of the acute patient. They can give important and nonspecific information to help choose an appropriate time for additional imaging, especially CT.[2–5] Traditionally, all patients suspected of having acute mesenteric ischemia underwent immediate diagnostic angiography,[6] whereas in case of peritoneal signs and abnormal lactic acid levels immediate surgery should be required.[6] The role of angiography and interventional vascular procedures in the management of acute mesenteric ischemia could be considered effective in case of early diagnosis of arterial embolism or thrombotic occlusion (**Fig. 1**) and in the absence of intestinal severe injury. Several factors have been claimed to contribute to a lethal outcome for acute mesenteric ischemia:[7] diagnosis after development of intestinal infarction, progression from ischemia to

infarction after correction of the cardiac or vascular cause, and the presence of nonocclusive intestinal ischemia of late stage with infarction of the bowel.

MDCT actually could be considered a comprehensive imaging method to evaluate either mesenteric vasculature status or small bowel appearance,[8–19] both of which have to be evaluated for a diagnosis of ischemia before development of intestinal necrosis and infarction. This article discusses the MDCT findings from ischemia to infarction of the small bowel related to arterial etiology, nonocclusive vascular disease, and impaired venous drainage intestinal injuries.

SMALL BOWEL INJURY FROM ARTERIAL ETIOLOGY

For an effective comprehension of the intestinal manifestations as consequence of whatever injury, it is essential to know and consider in the

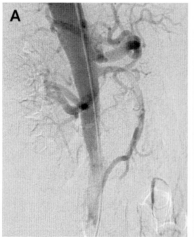
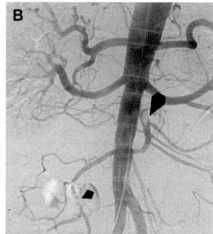
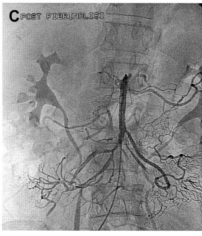

Fig. 1. Superior mesenteric arteriogram shows occlusion of the superior mesenteric artery (*A*) proximally and at the level of the ileal branches (*arrowheads* in *B*) and the normal opacification of the vessels after fibrinolysis (*C*).

diagnostic evaluation of the imaging findings that the intestine is something "alive" and "responding" to the pathologic event. The activity of two layers of smooth muscle cells effects contractions of the small bowel,[20] which is richly innervated by elements of the autonomic nervous system.[20] Within the wall of the intestine lie neurons, nerve endings, and receptors of the enteric nervous system, which structure tend to be concentrated in several plexi.[20] Extrinsic innervation of the small intestine is supplied by the vagus nerve and nervous fibers from the celiac and superior mesenteric ganglia.[20] Between contractions, pressure inside the lumen of the small intestine is approximately equal to the intra-abdominal pressure.[20] When the musculature contracts, the lumen is occluded partially or totally, and the pressure increases.[20]

The effect that any contraction could have on the intestinal contents depends on the state of the musculature above and below the point of the contraction.[20] If a contraction is not coordinated with the activity above and below, intestinal content is displaced proximally and distally during the contraction and may flow back during relaxation.[20] This activity mixes and locally circulates the contents.[20] Such contractions seem to divide the bowel into segments.[20] The peristaltic response could be considered as a high coordinated contractile activity that is propulsive in function,[20] causing net aboral transit.[20] Altered small bowel intestinal motility that results in delayed transit frequently accompanies a variety of diseases and clinical conditions.[20] The most common alteration in motility is the so-called transient ileus or apparent paralysis of the small bowel, which is sometimes appreciable after abdominal surgery and in the case of intra-abdominal inflammation.[20]

Although the peristaltic reflex depends on an intact enteric nervous system, another reflex, the so-called "intestine-intestinal reflex," depends on extrinsic neural connections.[20] If an area of the bowel is grossly distended, contractile activity in the rest of the bowel is inhibited.[20] The small bowel is under the influence of higher center of the nervous system; however, many circulating and endogenously released chemicals may alter intestinal motility.[20] Considering the entire pathophysiology of the visceral circulation, the splanchnic area receives approximately 25% of the cardiac output in a resting person, so the event caused in different disease conditions could be correlated to this fact.[21]

Because the pathophysiologic changes in the splanchnic area may contribute in greater part to the development of critical illness, it should be important to try to understand the underlying process and the visceral reactions to hypotension, hemorrhage, and sepsis.[21] The gastrointestinal vascular system is built up from circuits coupled in parallel, each of which consists of sections coupled in series.[21,22] These circuits are directed to the different layers of the gastrointestinal wall.[21] Anatomically, the resistance vessels correspond with the arterioles, so that most of the resistance to blood flow and the pressure drop over the circuit takes place in this segment.[21] The balance between the pre- and the postcapillary sphincters—with the term "sphincter" here used as a functional and not anatomic entity—determines the mean hydrostatic capillary pressure and the direction and the magnitude of any net fluid movement across the capillary wall.[21] In the capillary, the important exchange of fluid and metabolites takes place.[21] The major part of the regional blood volume is contained in the capacitance segment, which corresponds to the veins and larger venulae.[21] The blood directed to the splanchnic organs has to pass two capillary beds (primary organ and hepatic capillary bed) before returning to the heart.[21]

To maintain a consistent force for blood in the secondary portal circulation, the venous pressure of the first capillary bed (eg, the small bowel) has to be high;[21] however, the balance between the pre- and postcapillary resistance allows a mean hydrostatic capillary pressure to prevent net movements of fluid over the capillary walls.[21,23] This fact is important because the huge capillary bed of the viscera and the much higher capillary permeability in this capillaries could create a potential for significant fluid losses.[21] The gastrointestinal reaction after sympathetic vasoconstrictor nerve stimulation differs from other anatomic districts: in the gut, activation of sympathetic nerve induces a prompt vasoconstriction that subsides after a minute despite ongoing nerve activation.[21,24] After a couple of minutes, a steady-state situation is reached for the remainder of the nerve activation time, whereas blood flow is slightly reduced and the resistance to blood flow is increased only slightly with respect to the prestimulation period.[21] This effect is caused by the gastrointestinal autoregulatory escape from the response to the sympathetic nerve stimulation.[21]

After cessation of the nerve stimulation, there is a paradoxic hyperemic response, the reactive hyperemia.[21] Pathophysiology of the visceral circulation during hypovolemia and other critical illness conditions depends on the natural reactions of the vascular smooth cells of the visceral vessels and on the influence of the systemic parts of the body exerted on the visceral vasculature and its smooth cells.[21] The natural response of the smooth muscle is to relax when tension is reduced and to contract when the tension is increased.[21,25] After a self-monitoring process, changes in the vasculature tend to guarantee a more or less constant flow, even if blood pressure varies.[21]

The pathologic manifestations of the intestinal injury from diminished blood arterial mesenteric flow as sequential findings from correlated consequential events were noted more than one century ago by Litten[26] with his studies on dogs. Litten[26,27] found that the ligation of superior mesenteric artery resulted in death within 12 to 48 hours of all 40 dogs, accompanied by vomiting, bloody diarrhea, and fever. The immediate effects of typing the superior mesenteric artery presented as follows: all pulsation disappeared and the bowel became blue-white and spastic, with collapsed arteries and prominent veins.[26,27] Contractions increased initially but eventually disappeared; after some hours, the loops became relaxed and distended.[26,27]

Correlation between pathologic signs and known imaging findings of intestinal vascular disease from arterial mesenteric occlusion or low-flow state in a multi-stage progression scheme has been reported, based on the experience in emergency acute abdominal conditions at our institution (Table 1).[15]

Because the early reaction of the intestine to an injury seems to be regulated by a neurogenic answer, in acute abdominal conditions the early findings could be related to spastic and hypotonic reflex ileus as primarily reactions of the intestine.[5] Acute abdomen conditions caused by a reduced delivery of oxygen as the result of inadequate blood flow to the small intestine could have as initial appearance the evidence of spastic, collapsed small intestinal loops, with the corresponding "gasless" abdomen. "Gasless" indicates the condition in which there is no gas inside the intestine (differentiating it from other conditions, such as

Table 1
Schematic spectrum of injury progression in vascular disease of the small bowel from arterial etiology. The imaging findings in the various stages could be recognized, predominantly with CT, which offers a comprehensive view of the intestine, the mesenteric vasculature, and the entire abdominal compartment

SPASTIC REFLEX ILEUS

I STAGE

HYPOTONIC ILEUS

II STAGE

Reperfusion   No Reperfusion

III STAGE   IV STAGE: INFARCTION

HEALING

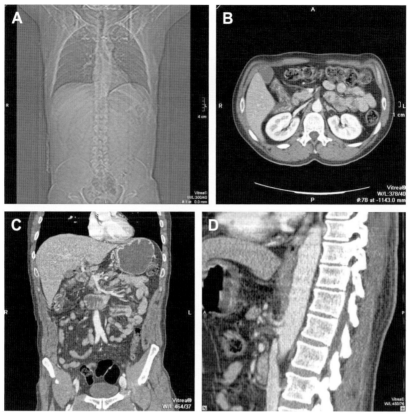

Fig. 2. A 42-year-old man with acute abdominal pain. MDCT scout view (A) and axial and coronal scans (B, C) show the evidence of a "spastic reflex ileus" with the collapsed entire small bowel and the evidence of parietal thrombosis of the superior mesenteric artery (SMA) at the origin with stenosis of the lumen (D). No diminished parietal enhancement of the small intestine and no alterations in appearance of the intestinal layers are noted. These findings could be considered the early "phase" of the vascular injury from arterial diminished blood flow.

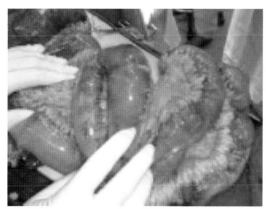

Fig. 3. Surgical finding of a "paper-thin" intestinal infarction from occlusion of the superior mesenteric artery. (Courtesy of Giovanni Bartone, MD, Naples, Italy.)

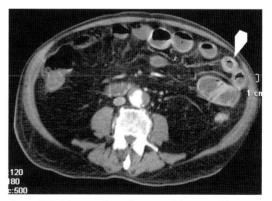

Fig. 4. MDCT scan of an 81-year-old man with acute abdominal pain after atrial fibrillation. The examination does not show a significantly reduced caliber of the distal branches of the superior mesenteric artery, whereas in some small bowel segments at the left abdominal quadrant there is hyperdensity of the wall (arrowhead) (III stage of ischemia). The patient recovered without sequelae.

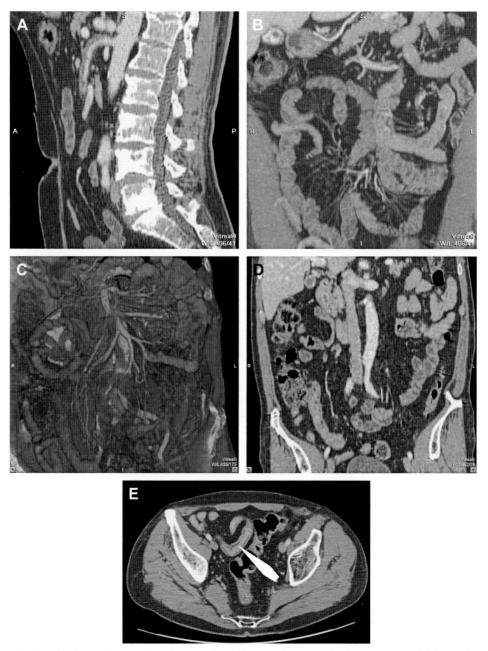

Fig. 5. Extensive dilation and concentric thrombosis of the superior mesenteric artery in a middle-aged patient. MDCT scan shows the appearance of the artery (*A*, sagittal view) with extensive thrombosis extended to the distal ileal branches (*B*, coronal view), which is also evident at the volumetric reconstruction (*C*). Distal small bowel loops are characterized by reperfusion findings, with slight hyperdensity of the mucosa and submucosal edema (*D*) (III stage). Note that distal ileal loops in the pelvis presented hyperdense fluid in the lumen (blood) (*E, arrowhead*).

"gasless" because of the absence of air in the lumen due to completely fluid-distended loops—mechanical ileus—or the presence of massive ascites in patients who have hepatopathy.[5]

Using MDCT, when we have the chance to scan the patient at the beginning of the disease (stage I), we can appreciate the evidence of collapsed small intestine that presents as normal (or in some cases hyperemic) enhancement of the wall (**Fig. 2**). Performing MDCT examination in the arterial and venous phases using optimal examination protocol, short back-reconstruction interval, and adequate

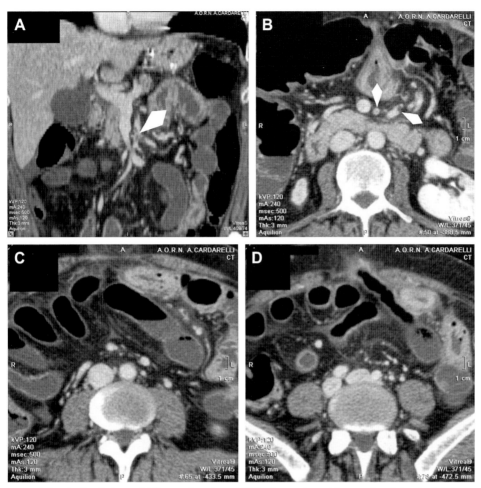

Fig. 6. Acute abdominal pain in a middle-aged patient. MDCT shows the evidence of endoluminal defects of opacification in the superior mesenteric artery (*A, B, arrowheads*). Note the presence of different appearance of the small intestine: some loops are distended, predominantly by air, but the endoluminal stasis seems to be growing up. Some others are characterized by intramural hemorrhage and edema (reperfusion injury, III stage) (*C, D*).

peripheral venous access to administer intravenous contrast medium at 3.5 mL/sec at least, a great evaluation of the mesenteric vasculature could be obtained, together with an excellent view of the entire intestine morphology, conditions, and parietal enhancement.

The hypotonic ileus follows a reflex spastic ileus; at this phase (stage II) the small bowel loops appear distended by air with loss of tone[15] and the "paper thin" wall could be appreciated. Usually, MDCT indicates that the wall enhancement could be normal or decreased. From stage II, if the ischemia persists long enough without reperfusion, the disease may progress to infarction (**Fig. 3**).[15]

When MDCT examination indicates the presence of air-dilated small bowel loops, occlusion of the superior mesenteric artery or a diminished caliber of the opacified vessel in a patient with suggestive clinical history for mesenteric ischemia

could give us the opportunity to diagnose intestinal ischemia, whereas in the absence of vessel abnormalities and nonspecific clinical data, an alternative diagnostic hypothesis should be considered. Per our personal experience, when the appearance of the small intestine is altered and the clinical symptoms suggest intestinal ischemia, low-flow state condition must be considered strongly.

In Litten's experience, after the phase of "spasticity" and "hypotonia," 8 to 10 hours later frank hemorrhage occurred. Autopsy of the bowel from the duodeno-jejunal flexure to the transverse colon revealed that it was dark red and soaked in bloody edema.[26,27] The serosal coat was raised in blebs, and there was bleeding into the muscular layers, whereas the mucosa was swollen by a massive secretion of sero-sanguineous fluid.[26,27] This appearance is identical to that later described by

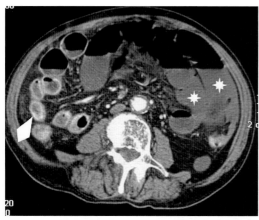

Fig. 7. An 85-year-old patient affected by cardiopathy and arteriosclerosis who referred several recent episodes of moderate abdominal pain underwent MDCT for acute abdominal pain. CT scans show the evidence of defect of opacification of the distal branches of the superior mesenteric artery and the evidence of marked dilation with parietal thickening, endoluminal fluid, and absence of enhancement of the small bowel at the left quadrant (*white asterisks*) (IV stage). At right, some segments of the small intestine presented as hyperdensity of the wall from III stage disease (*arrowhead*).

other authors in human subjects after mesenteric embolus.[27–29] Additional studies conducted in the 1960s to evaluate the effects of acute occlusion of the superior mesenteric artery confirmed Litten's observation, attesting that 3 to 4 hours after an initial reaction of spasm, the tone disappeared and the bowel became cyanotic and edematous, with increased swelling in the next few hours.[30] The bowel became progressively

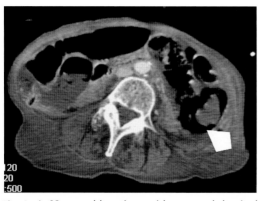

Fig. 8. A 92-year-old patient with acute abdominal pain was diagnosed as having intestinal infarction from arterial etiology (IV stage). This figure shows the presence of massive intestinal infarction with marked parietal pneumatosis at the left quadrant (*arrowhead*).

damaged with evidence of necrosis.[27,30] Turbid fluid also was present in the peritoneal cavity, and mesenteric pneumatosis was apparent.[30] Acute microscopic changes of the bowel wall during and after superior mesenteric artery occlusion have been described in dogs;[31,32] degenerative changes in the villi seem to occur 30 minutes after vessel occlusion, but marked alterations occurred later. Two hours after superior mesenteric artery occlusion, intracellular changes were appreciated in the mucosal cells, with various damage extension progressively seen after 3 to 5 hours later and marked alterations and intracellular edema present in the crypts.[32]

In addition to the injuries caused by ischemia, a reperfusion component of tissue injury could be evident after the ischemic event, when reperfusion of the involved intestine occurs.[21] When reperfusion occurs, depending on degree of microvascular wall damage, blood plasma, contrast medium, or erythrocytes may extravasate through the disrupted vascular wall and mucosa, causing wall thickening and fluid filling the lumen.[33] At this stage III, MDCT examination could give us information regarding the mesenteric arterial vasculature and the small bowel wall appearance (**Figs. 4–6**).

If reperfusion damage is not relevant, healing of the involved intestine could be appreciated, whereas if the vascular disease caused severe nonreversible injuries, infarction can develop as a late stage (stage IV) of the disease progression (**Fig. 7**). On CT, small bowel infarction presents as evidence of absent enhancement of the intestinal wall, presence of pneumatosis, and free air in the peritoneum if perforation has occurred (**Figs. 8 and 9**). The importance of considering mesenteric vessels opacification could be secondary to the evidence of the intestinal signs of necrosis at this stage. **Table 1** presents a proposed scheme based on the pathophysiologic progression of events of the vascular disease of the small intestine from mesenteric arterial occlusion/low-flow states.

In the past, most of the reports of the scientific literature in diagnostic radiology considered intestinal ischemia as a consequence not only of arterial etiology disease but also of other causes (eg, intestinal obstruction). Reaction of the intestine seems to be different in the various causes, and differences in changes of the parietal wall could be noted and recognized with imaging methodology if the pathologic mechanism that offers the different feature and findings is known.

In our experience we tried to correlate the pathologic data with the imaging findings[15] and noted that as the progressive histopathologic changes occur—from the damage to the epithelium to

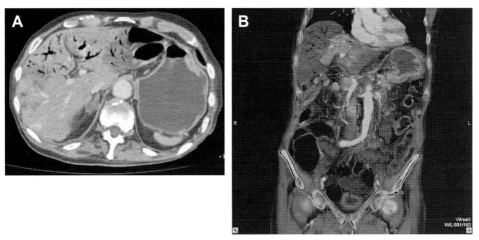

Fig. 9. Late stage of disease from arterial etiology. MDCT shows the evidence of portal, mesenteric, and parietal pneumatosis in a massive infarction of the intestine (A, B).

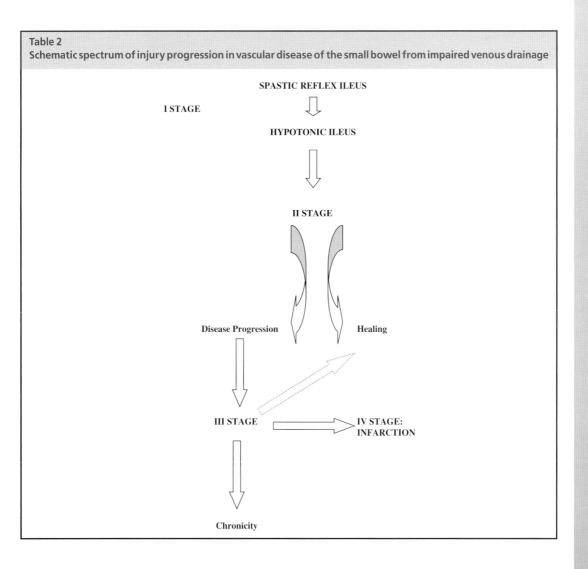

Table 2
Schematic spectrum of injury progression in vascular disease of the small bowel from impaired venous drainage

SPASTIC REFLEX ILEUS

I STAGE

HYPOTONIC ILEUS

II STAGE

Disease Progression   Healing

III STAGE   IV STAGE:
                   INFARCTION

Chronicity

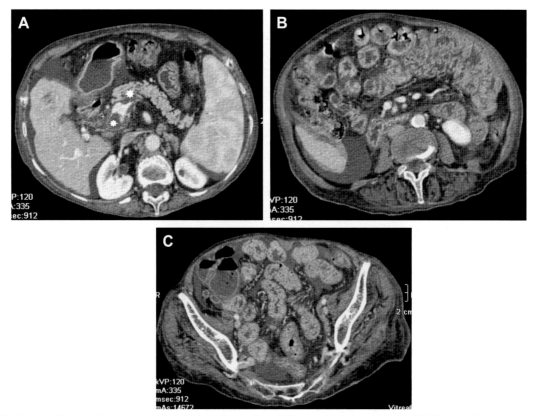

Fig. 10. An 85-year-old patient with hepatopathy and portal-mesenteric thrombosis. MDCT scans show the evidence of extensive defect of opacification within the lumen of the spleno-portal trunk (*A, asterisks*) and the appearance of the intestine, characterized by parietal thickening and transmural hyperdensity caused by submucosal hemorrhage (*B, C*).

inflammation, edema, and hemorrhage into the submucosa and the late stage of intestinal vascular disease (infarction), in which necrosis of the intestine is evident—the imaging findings[15] could be considered in a four-stage classification and appreciated with effectiveness by MDCT examinations (**Table 1**).

SMALL BOWEL INJURY OF VENOUS ORIGIN

Thrombosis of the mesenteric vein may occur in acute and chronic forms.[34] Patients with the chronic form can be symptomatic for weeks or months and require medical treatment or improve spontaneously because of formation of collateral vessels.[34] Different from acute arterial mesenteric disease, the acute form of mesenteric venous injury is characterized by a slow evolution of days or weeks before presenting with increased and persistent abdominal pain.[34] Mesenteric venous thrombosis is frequently observed in patients affected by cirrhosis or portal hypertension, but it can be primary.[15] Other conditions, such as

coagulation disorders, polycytemia, high platelet levels, and systemic disease (eg, lupus erythematosus) and the use of estrogen-progesteronic therapy may represent risks factors for development of mesenteric thrombosis.[15,35,36]

Although it is not rare to observe mesenteric thrombosis in a clinical radiologic practice and to appreciate the corresponding imaging findings from related intestinal disease, especially in patients who have hepatopathy, signs of intestinal infarction from impaired venous drainage are uncommon. Because of the features of the small bowel segments affected by mesenteric venous drainage disease, a "dead" intestinal segment may not be immediately distinguished from a "highly involved" one by the disease. The pathophysiology of acute mesenteric venous occlusion was studied by Polk[37] in 1964 while studying an experimental model of disease in dogs, when he noted rapid fluid sequestration and capillary rupture that resulted in submucosal and subserosal hemorrhage and evidence of sero-sanguineous ascites. Although there are differences in collateral

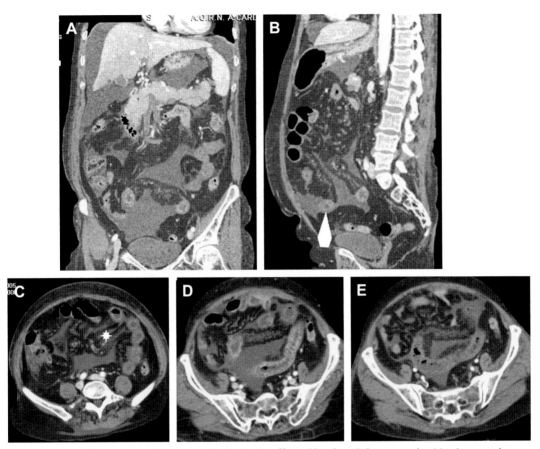

Fig. 11. A 60-year-old patient with acute abdominal pain affected by chronic hepatopathy. Massive portal-mesenteric thrombosis is evident (*A*) at the MDCT examination. Target sign with submucosal edema and hyperdensity of the mucosa (*B, arrowhead*) and the mesenteric engorgement (*C, asterisk*) are evident. Note the similar appearance of the intestine in the pelvis (*D*) at a following control 3 days after the first examination, after medical therapy (*E*), with persistence of the symptomatology.

flow of the canine intestine, the results in human beings are similar once vascular occlusion occurs.[38] The thrombosed veins cause congestion, swelling, and hemorrhage of the bowel wall, with fluid flowing out from the bowel and mesentery into the peritoneal cavity.[34,39,40] Venous occlusion causes mucosal edema and punctate hemorrhage that progress to widespread hemorrhages within minutes.[41] Progression of the thrombosis and inadequate collateral circulation leads to infarction of the jejunum and the ileum.[42] Necrosis and sloughing of the mucosa occurred in canine experiments at 180 minutes, whereas serosal hemorrhage and infarction occurred in 3 hours.[34,41] In clinical observation of humans, the time course is different—longer—because of the differences in collateral circulation.[34]

From a diagnostic imaging point of view, because the symptomatology of the impaired mesenteric venous drainage is less acute than in arterial ischemic disease, visualizing the initial phase is not easy or common.[15] Reaction of the small intestine to the mesenteric venous occlusion at the beginning also could be characterized by spasticity without bowel distension.[15] Because of the slow process underlying the impaired venous drainage disease, visualization of the subsequent hypotonic ileus could be difficult, with the findings masked by progressive intramural and mesenteric edema.[15] Correlation between pathologic signs and known imaging findings of intestinal vascular disease from impaired venous drainage in a multi-stage progression scheme was also attempted based on the experience in our Institution (**Table 2**).[15]

With MDCT, if a patient with an acute abdominal condition and evidence of superior mesenteric venous thrombosis has a spastic intestine not distended by gas or fluid, we can presume to have done the scan in the early stage I of disease. If during CT scan we note mesenteric vein occlusion and distension of the small intestine by air, we

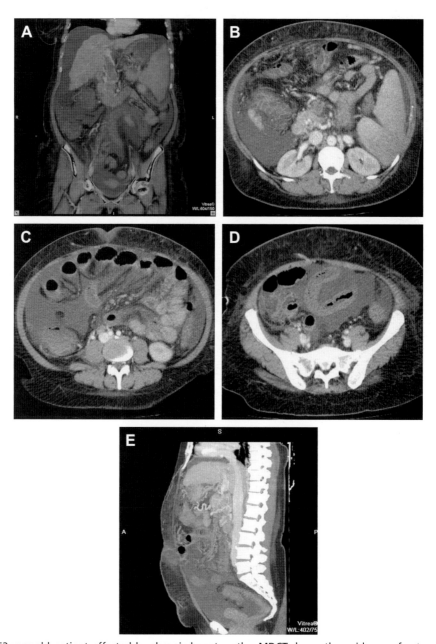

Fig. 12. A 52-year-old patient affected by chronic hepatopathy. MDCT shows the evidence of extensive portal-mesenteric thrombosis (A) and diffuse findings of intestinal injury from impaired venous drainage, particularly appreciable at the level of the right colon (B, C), whereas in the pelvis some ileal segments are affected by II/III stage of disease with overlapped thickening from chronic affection (D). Note also the presence of portal collateral circulation (E).

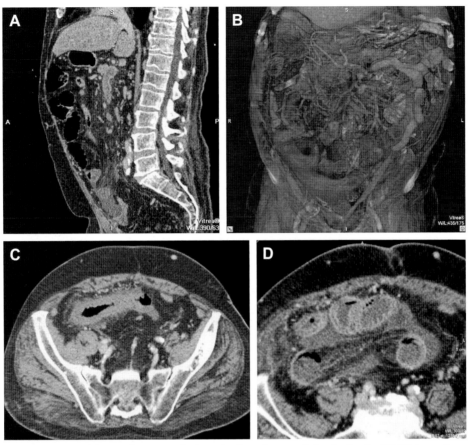

Fig. 13. Elederly patient with portal-mesenteric thrombosis and acute abdominal pain. MDCT shows the evidence of occlusion of the portal-mesenteric axis (A) and the presence of diffuse findings from stage III disease affecting the intestine (B), particularly the distal ileum (C). After few days of medical therapy because of persistence of the symptoms, the patient underwent another CT examination that confirmed the evidence of marked disease of the distal ileum with evidence of higher engorgement of the mesentery and presence of some bubbles of parietal pneumatosis (D). Because of the worsening of the clinical conditions, he underwent surgery that confirmed the evidence of a segmental infarction of the small intestine.

can presume that the patient is in the late stage I of disease. The intestinal wall in these cases could appear "normal" and have a regular appearance on enhancement. Although results of a patient who undergoes CT examination at the beginning of intestinal vascular disease may show impaired venous drainage, it is more common to find signs of more advanced disease.

When mesenteric venous occlusion progresses, intravascular volume increases, hydrostatic pressure rises, and arterial blood flows into capillaries and venules of the bowel and mesentery.[33,43] This causes extravasation of plasma, contrast material, and red blood cells in the fenestrations of the arterocapillary endothelium into the submucosa (Fig. 10).[43] This appearance is similar to features of reperfused ischemia.[43]

Imaging findings at stage II are related to bowel wall thickness, intramural hemorrhage, and submucosal edema.[15] With MDCT the imaging findings are related to the appearance of the intestine involved by disease from impaired venous drainage, with typical alternating different density layers ("target" sign): hyperdense mucosa caused by surface hemorrhage and ulceration and hypodense edematous submucosa (Fig. 11).[15]

This stage of disease may be reversible because deeper layers of the intestinal wall are preserved.[15] A complete healing of the mesenteric vein thrombosis can be obtained by medical therapy. Healing of the affected segment may lead to circumferential granulation tissue formation in response to the parietal damage;[15] however, if the disease progresses, chronicity of the affection or progression to intestinal infarction may be observed.[15] Persistence of a venous thrombosis leads to mesenteric vascular engorgement and edema with formation of venous collateral vessels.[44]

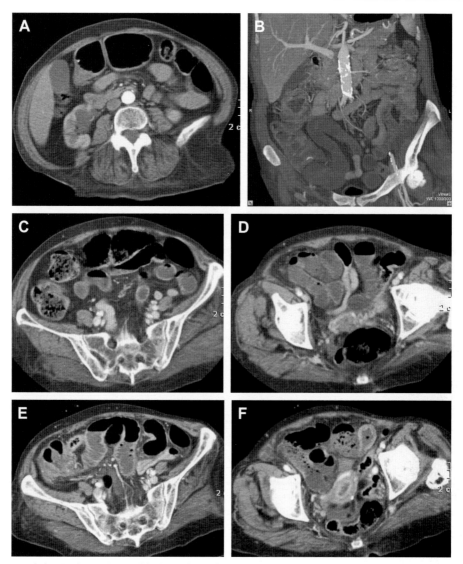

Fig. 14. Acute abdominal pain in an elderly cardiopathic patient. MDCT scan revealed the relatively reduced caliber of the superior mesenteric artery (A). The coronal view (B) shows the presence of different patterns of appearance of the small intestine: some loops are distended and some others are collapsed (C, D); however, there is no sign of mechanical obstruction. A first diagnosis of disease from low-flow state was attempted. Because the abdominal symptoms persisted, the following control 2 days later showed the presence of more distinguished pattern of III stage in some small intestine loops in the pelvis (E), with decreased enhancement from segmental infarction confirmed at surgery of some ileal segments (F) distended by fluid with signs of endoluminal stasis.

At stage III of disease, MDCT may reveal evidence of mesenteric thrombosis, collateral circulation, thickened small bowel wall, peritoneal fluid, and mesenteric engorgement (Fig. 12).

Progression to intestinal infarction at stage IV of disease is characterized by extensive submucosal hemorrhage and edema.[15] When the tension in the extravascular compartment of the submucosa increases, the arterial supply could be compromised, with decreased enhancement of the mucosa.[43] The tissue tension may cause complete failure of the arterial supply because of blood flow stasis.[43] Cyanosis may lead to bowel wall rupture, with consequent necrosis and peritonitis.[15] With MDCT, findings of intestinal infarction at late stage IV from impaired venous drainage are related to

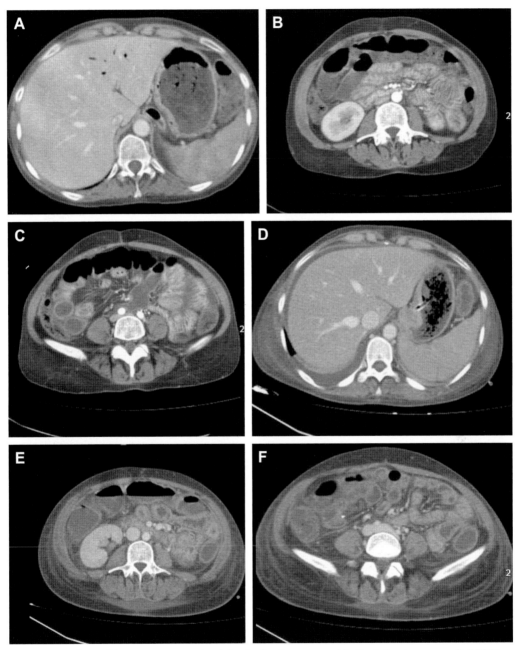

Fig. 15. Young patient with postpartum acute abdominal pain recovered in the intensive vare unit. MDCT examination showed the evidence of intrahepatic portal pneumatosis (A). The appearance of the intestine was similar to that of injury from reperfusion (B, C). There was no evidence of mesenteric arterial/venous disease. The patient presented with marked electrolyte imbalance. The following control 3 days later showed moderate improvement of the intestinal reperfusion findings with slight remission of the symptomatology (D–F).

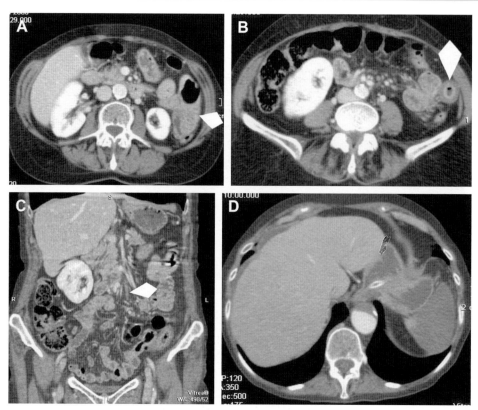

Fig. 16. A 74-year-old patient underwent MDCT examination for acute abdominal pain. The presence of some small bowel loops affected by reperfusion findings (A, B, arrowheads) and the lack of opacification of an ileal branch of the superior mesenteric artery (C, arrowhead) were missed in the report. Because of the remission of the abdominal pain, the patient was dismissed few days later. Thirteen days after the first acute event, the patient presented again to our institution for acute abdominal pain. The MDCT showed findings of a dramatic progression of the vascular disease from alteration in blood supply, with evidence of splenic (D) and right renal infarction (E). The presence of the superior mesenteric artery occlusion was confirmed and well evident on coronal view (F). The small intestine appeared distended by fluid, with absence of parietal enhancement in most part of the ileum from late-stage ischemia (G).

evidence of mesenteric vein occlusion, peritoneal fluid, marked wall thickening, lack of enhancement, and intramural or portal-mesenteric pneumatosis (Fig. 13).

SUMMARY

Intestinal ischemia of the small bowel presents important diagnostic questions to be answered in emergency situations. Although some suggestive findings could be appreciated with basic imaging methods (eg, ultrasound, abdominal radiography), MDCT as a modern noninvasive imaging method could be effective in evaluating intestinal disease caused by superior mesenteric artery or vein occlusion and diagnosing ischemia from low-flow states in cases of alteration of arterial vessel caliber and suggestive clinical findings.

Intestinal small bowel ischemia from low-flow states could present different imaging patterns depending on the acuteness and duration of the reduced blood supply (Fig. 14). It should be also stressed the concept that the exclusive note to the mesenteric vessels could represent a great diagnostic limit if a correct and comprehensive evaluation of the small bowel appearance is not done (Fig. 15). Looking at the features of the parietal layers and the enhancement and morphology of the loops—collapsed or distended by air or fluid—with knowledge of the pathologic mechanism underlying the changes from the "normality" (Fig. 16) could be helpful in making a correct, prompt, and effective diagnosis of intestinal ischemia or disease from impaired venous drainage, which is important for management of the patient.

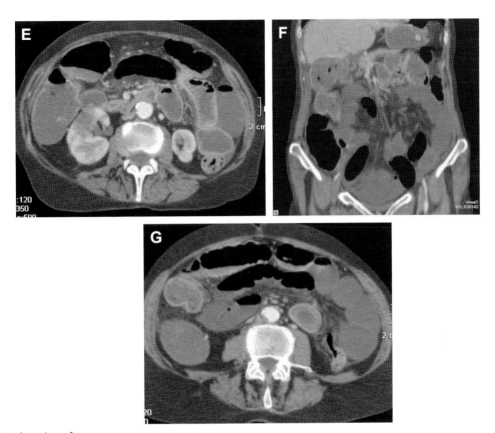

Fig. 16. (continued)

REFERENCES

1. Turnage RH, Myers SI. Pathophysiology. In: Longo WE, Peterson GJ, Jacobs DL, editors. Intestinal ischemia disorders. St.Louis (MO): Quality Medical Publishing, Inc; 1998. p. 17–49.

2. Wadman M, Syk I, Elmståhl B, et al. Abdominal plain film findings in acute ischemic bowel disease differ with age. Acta Radiol 2006;47(3):238–43.

3. Hayes R. Abdominal pain: general imaging strategies. Eur Radiol 2004;14(Suppl 4):L123–37.

4. Dietrich CF, Jedrzejczyk M, Ignee A. Sonographic assessment of splanchnic arteries and the bowel wall. Eur J Radiol 2007;64(2):202–12.

5. Grassi R, Di Mizio R, Pinto A, et al. Serial plain abdominal film findings in the assessment of acute abdomen: spastic ileus, hypotonic ileus, mechanical ileus and paralytic ileus. Radiol Med 2004; 108(1–2):56–70.

6. Hagspiel KD, Angle JF, Spinosa DJ, et al. Angiography: diagnosis and therapeutics. In: Longo WE, Peterson GJ, Jacobs DL, editors. Intestinal ischemia disorders. St.Louis (MO): Quality Medical Publishing, Inc; 1998. p. 105–54.

7. Boley SJ, Sammartano RJ, Brandt LJ. Historical perspective. In: Longo WE, Peterson GJ, Jacobs DL, editors. Intestinal ischemia disorders. St.Louis (MO): Quality Medical Publishing, Inc; 1998. p. 1–15.

8. Fleischmann D. Multiple detector-row CT angiography of the renal and mesenteric vessels. Eur J Radiol 2003;45(Suppl 1):S79–87.

9. Haage P, Krings T, Schmitz-Rode T. Nontraumatic vascular emergencies: imaging and intervention in acute venous occlusion. Eur Radiol 2002;12(11): 2627–43.

10. Fishman EK, Horton KM. The increasing impact of multidetector row computed tomography in clinical practice. Eur J Radiol 2007;62(Suppl):1–13.

11. Shih MC, Hagspiel KD. CTA and MRA in mesenteric ischemia. Part 1. Role in diagnosis and differential diagnosis. AJR Am J Roentgenol 2007;188(2): 452–61.

12. Shih MC, Angle JF, Leung DA, et al. CTA and MRA in mesenteric ischemia. Part 2. Normal findings and complications after surgical and endovascular treatment. AJR Am J Roentgenol 2007;188(2):462–71.

13. Kirkpatrick ID, Kroeker MA, Greenberg HM. Biphasic CT with mesenteric CT angiography in the

evaluation of acute mesenteric ischemia: initial experience. Radiology 2003;229(1):91–8.

14. Hellinger JC. Evaluating mesenteric ischemia with multidetector-row CT angiography. Tech Vasc Interv Radiol 2004;7(3):160–6.

15. Romano S, Lassandro F, Scaglione M, et al. Ischemia and infarction of the small bowel and colon: spectrum of imaging findings. Abdom Imaging 2006;31(3):277–92.

16. Bradbury MS, Kavanagh PV, Bechtold RE, et al. Mesenteric venous thrombosis: diagnosis and noninvasive imaging. Radiographics 2002;22(3): 527–41.

17. Gaven K, Acunaay B. Multidetector computed tomography angiography of the abdomen. Eur J Radiol 2004;52(1):44–55.

18. Hong SS, Kim AY, Byun JH, et al. MDCT of small-bowel disease: value of 3D imaging. AJR Am J Roentgenol 2006;187(5):1212–21.

19. Levi AD. Mesenteric ischemia. Radiol Clin North Am 2007;45(3):593–9.

20. Weisbrodt NW. Motility of the small intestine. In: Johnson LR, editor. Gastrointestinal physiology. 7th edition. Philadelphia: Mosby Elsevier; 2007. p. 41–7.

21. Haglund UH. Pathophysiology of the visceral circulation. In: Geroulakos G, Cherry KJ Jr, editors. Disease of the visceral circulation. London: Arnold, Hodder Headline Group; 2002. p. 24–38.

22. Folkow B. Regional adjustments of intestinal blood flow. Gastroenterology 1967;52:423–32.

23. Folkow B, Leewis DH, Lundgren O, et al. The effect of the sympathetic vasoconstrictor fibres on the distribution of capillary blood flow in the intestine. Acta Physiol Scand 1964;61:458–66.

24. Folkow B, Lewis DH, Lundgren O, et al. The effect of graded vasoconstrictor fibre stimulation on the intestinal resistance and capacitance vessels. Acta Physiol Scand 1964;61:445–57.

25. Johnson PC, Hanson KM. Effect of arterial pressure on arterial and venous resistance of intestine. J Appl Physiol 1962;17:503–8.

26. Litten M. Uber die folgen des verschkusses der arteria meseraica superior. Virchows Arch. Pathol Anat J 1875;63:289–312 [German].

27. Marston A. Laboratory studies of intestinal ischemia. In: Vascular disease of the gastrointestinal tract. 2nd edition. Baltimore (MD): Williams and Wilkins; 1986. p. 30–51.

28. Hertzler AE. Surgical pathology of the peritoneum. Philadelphia: JB Lippincott; 1935.

29. Boyd W. Surgical pathology. 6th edition. Philadelphia: WB Saunders; 1947. p. 565.

30. Marston A. Causes of death in mesenteric arterial occlusion. Ann Surg 1963;58:952–60.

31. Ahonen J, Inberg MV, Jaaskelainen AJ, et al. Effect of oxygen ventilation in mesenteric arterial occlusion in dog. Scand J Gastroenterol 1972;7(1):9–16.

32. Aho AJ, Arstila AU, Ahonen J, et al. Ultrastructural alterations in ischaemic lesion of small intestinal mucosa in experimental superior mesenteric artery occlusion. Scand J Gastroenterol 1973;8(5): 439–47.

33. Chou CK, Mak CW, Tzeng WS, et al. CT of small bowel ischemia. Abdom Imaging 2004;29:18–22.

34. Laureano BA, Wade TP. Mesenteric venous disease. In: Longo WE, Peterson GJ, Jacobs DL, editors. Intestinal ischemia disorders. St. Louis (MO): Quality Medical Publishing, Inc; 1998. p. 207–19.

35. Jost CJ, Gloviczki P. Mesenteric vein thrombosis. In: Geroulakos G, Cherry KJ Jr, editors. Disease of the visceral circulation. London: Arnold, Hodder Headline Group; 2002. p. 145–57.

36. Kitchens CS. Evolution of our understanding of the pathophysiology of primary mesenteric venous thrombosis. Am J Surg 1992;163:346–8.

37. Polk HC. Experimental mesenteric vein occlusion. Am J Surg 1964;88:693–8.

38. Noer RJ. The blood vessels of the jejunum and ileum: a comparative study of man and certain laboratory animals. Am J Anat 1943;73:293–334.

39. Friedberg MJ, Polk HC Jr. Superior mesenteric arteriography in experimental mesenteric venous thrombosis. Radiology 1965;85:38–45.

40. Polk HC Jr. Experimental mesenteric venous occlusion. III. Diagnosis and treatment of induced mesenteric venous thrombosis. Ann Surg 1966;163: 432–44.

41. Macfadyen BV, Gliga L, Al-Kaisi NK, et al. Endoscopic and histologic correlates of intestinal ischemia in a canine model. Am Surg 1988;54:68–72.

42. Rhee RY, Gloviczki P, Mendonca CT, et al. Mesenteric venous thrombosis: still a lethal disease in the 1990's. J Vasc Surg 1994;20:688–97.

43. Chou CK. CT manifestation of bowel ischemia. AJR Am J Roentgenol 2002;178:87–91.

44. Kim JY, Ha HK, Byun JY, et al. J Comput Assist Tomogr. J Comput Assist Tomogr 1993;17:382–5.

Imaging of Ischemic Colitis

P. Taourel, MD, PhD[a],*, Sophie Aufort, MD[b], Samuel Merigeaud, MD[a],
Fernanda Curros Doyon, MD[a], Marine Devaux Hoquet, MD[a],
Eric Delabrousse, MD[c]

KEYWORDS
• Ischemia • Colitis • US • CT

Ischemic colitis accounts for more than half of all cases of gastrointestinal ischemia and constitutes between 1 per 2000 and 3 per 1000 acute hospital admission. It typically affects elderly patients, being a frequent cause of rectal bleeding, abdominal pain, and diarrhea.[1–3] The condition comprises a broad range of presentations, from mild forms to fulminant cases. From the histologic point of view and in terms of the severity and evolution of the process, two presentations of ischemic colitis have been described: a gangrenous form associated with transmural necrosis with a high mortality rate and a transient form with reversible lesions limited to the mucosa or submucosa, which benefits from conservative management. This article describes the epidemiology, physiology, and pathology of this underdiagnosed condition; reviews the clinical patterns of this disease, which constitute a key diagnostic point in patients who have a thickening of the colonic wall; and describes the ultrasound (US) and CT findings, pitfalls, and differential diagnoses of ischemic colitis. The value and limitations of US and CT at the different diagnostic stages is discussed: positive diagnosis, severity diagnosis, and etiologic diagnosis.

EPIDEMIOLOGY

Since it was described initially by Boley and colleagues[4] in 1963, ischemic injury to the colon is now recognized to manifest distinct clinical subtypes, which range in severity from transient segmental colopathy to fulminant gangrenous colitis.[5,6] Ischemic colitis can be divided into two main types. The first form is a spontaneous, self-limiting form and occurs days or weeks after the initial ischemic insult. Colitis normally resolves with conservative therapy, although there may be a stricture during recovery. Conversely, some patients develop a fulminant form of the disease with transmural gangrenous necrosis of the colon, which is fatal if not treated early. Management of ischemic colitis depends on the severity of the illness. Surgical intervention is indicated if there is peritonitis, transmural infarction, failure to respond to medical management, chronic symptomatic colitis, or strictures.

The incidence of colonic ischemia in the general population remains unknown. Studies to date have focused on the inpatient population, and it is likely that many cases of transient ischemic injury are left undiagnosed.[5] Furthermore, in clinical practice, many cases of colonic ischemia are misdiagnosed as inflammatory bowel disease.[6] Last, there may be confusion between ischemic colitis and pseudomembranous colitis because they may have the same endoscopic pattern. Ischemic colitis is a relatively common entity and because life expectancy is increasing, physicians will face this problem more often. It constitutes the most common form of ischemic injury to the gastrointestinal tract and the second most common cause of lower gastrointestinal bleeding.[7,8]

[a] Department of Imaging, CHU Montpellier, Hospital Lapeyronie, 371 Avenue du Doyen Gaston-Giraud, 34295 Montpellier Cedex 5, France
[b] Department of Imaging, CHU Montpellier, Hospital St Eloi, 80 Avenue Augustin Fliche, 34295 Montpellier Cedex 5, France
[c] Department of Imaging, CHU Besançon, Hospital Jean Minjoz, Radiologie A, 3 Bd Alexandre Fleming, 25030 Besançon, France
* Corresponding author.
E-mail address: p-taourel@chu-montpellier.fr (P. Taourel).

Radiol Clin N Am 46 (2008) 909–924
doi:10.1016/j.rcl.2008.06.003
0033-8389/08/$ – see front matter © 2008 Elsevier Inc. All rights reserved.

Vascular disease of the intestine may present different etiologies: bowel ischemia may be caused by arterial occlusive disease, venous occlusive disease, or nonocclusive ischemia resulting from low-flow state.[3,4] Arterial causes are related to thrombosis, stenosis attributable to atherosclerosis, or embolus; they may be a complication of interventional procedures (aortography, colectomy with ligation of inferior mesenteric artery, embolization of mesenteric artery, cardiac or aortic surgery) or may be localized to distal arteries in cases of radiation injury or systemic vasculitis disorders. Mesenteric vein thrombosis is related to pylephlebitis, hypercoagulable states, portal hypertension, pancreatitis, and small vessel disease. Nonthrombotic stenosis or occlusion of the mesenteric veins, such as mesenteric phlebosclerosis with calcifications in the small mesenteric veins, may also cause chronic ischemic colitis.[9] Low-flow state constituted the most common cause of ischemic colitis, with the development of colitis after the episode of low-flow has resolved in most cases.[10] Ischemic injury of the colon may also be related to administration of some medications or drugs, such as digitalis preparations, diuretics, catecholamines, estrogens, danazol, nonsteroidal anti-inflammatory drugs, neuroleptics, and laxatives.[10] Ischemic disease of the colon has also been noted as a consequence of cocaine abusers[10] or long-distance runners.[11] Last, ischemic colitis may develop proximally to colon obstruction.

Different clinical contexts make the diagnosis of ischemic colitis likely:

Cardiovascular disease, which is more often atherosclerosis than disease responsible for embolus, because inferior mesenteric artery emboli are uncommon; most emboli are too large to enter this narrow vessel.

Low-flow state in which vasoactive medications may have limited the flow to the ischemic segments or blunted the colon's ability to compensate for low blood flow.[2] In a monocentric retrospective study including 129 patients, 58% were receiving vasoactive medication.[2]

Chronic renal failure with hemodialysis, which constituted 20% of the patients who had ischemic colitis in the aforementioned study.[2]

Postsurgical patients. The two most common causes of postoperative ischemic colitis are cardiac surgery and aortic procedures since the improvement of the surgery of the colon. Ischemic colitis complicated 2.7% of a series of 1786 aortic reconstructions.[12] In a retrospective analysis of gastrointestinal emergencies after 3724 consecutive cardiac surgeries, ischemic colitis constituted the most frequent of the 1% of gastrointestinal complications.[13]

In young patients, causes of ischemic colitis include shock bowel trauma, hypercoagulable states, vasculitides such as systemic lupus erythematosus, polyarteritis nodosa, sickle cell disease, long-distance running, illicit drugs such as cocaine, or medicinal drugs such as oral contraceptives.

Usually, the ischemic event seems spontaneous and occurs without occlusion of a major blood vessel. In the colon, the overwhelming majority of cases present no identifiable cause, no iatrogenic injury, and no preceding problem; no precipitating episodes have been delineated.[10]

PHYSIOLOGY

Several factors seem to predispose the colon to ischemia, one being that the colon receives less blood flow than does the remainder of the gastrointestinal tract.[14] In fact, there is an extensive network of vessels within the bowel wall, arising from the vasa recta and vasa brevia in the mesenteric border of the bowel, which give rise to a microvascular plexus in the muscularis and submucosal layers; this microvasculature is less developed in the colon than in the thinner-walled small intestine.[10] A decrease in blood flow to 20% of the normal flow associated with small vessel disease (hypoxia), and reperfusion injury when the blood flow is reestablished are involved in the constitution of an ischemic colitis.[15,16] The reperfusion lesions are the likely determining factors in ischemic colitis with the colonic blood flow usually returned to normal by the time of clinical presentation. This phenomenon explains why mesenteric angiography is generally not contributive in ischemic colitis. The colonic mucosal changes are primarily attributable to the sudden restoration of blood flow through vasculature, with leaky capillaries brought about by superoxides. There are two particularly exposed areas: the Griffiths point at the splenic flexure at the junction between the superior mesenteric artery vascularization and the inferior mesenteric vascularization, and the Sudeck point in the left colon at the junction between the inferior mesenteric artery vascularization and the hypogastric artery. Ischemic proctosigmoiditis remains a rare entity because of the abundant collateral blood supply that is located within the pelvis and perineum. When this entity occurs, an identifiable precipitating factor is often identified;[17] for example, division of the superior rectal artery distal to the Sudeck's point may lead to rectal ischemia in the remaining rectosigmoid following sigmoidectomy.[18] The pathogenesis of right-side colonic involvement in patients who have chronic renal failure on hemodialysis has been implicated because of repeated hypotensive episodes that led to vasoconstriction of the vasa recta in the right colon.[19]

PATHOLOGY

Colonoscopy is classically the investigation of choice, enabling direct visualization of the mucosa and taking a biopsy.[3] Colonoscopy may show hemorrhagic nodules (representing submucosal bleeding) or the presence of a single linear ulcer running longitudinally (colonic single-stripe sign) mainly in the left side of the colon in mild ischemic colitis.[3,20,21] The histopathologic manifestations of ischemic colitis are mucosal necrosis and ulcerations, submucosal edema and hemorrhage, or transmural infarction. Mucosal damage is reversible, occurring as a self-limited condition, whereas necrosis of the muscle layer can lead to the development of a fibrotic stricture or to severe sepsis and perforation.

Overdistension of the colon at colonoscopy may cause high intraluminal pressure, however, which could exacerbate ischemic damage[22] and is particularly dangerous in cases of severe colitis with a risk for perforation. Endoscopic biopsy often cannot reveal the extension of ischemic injury into the colonic wall because the biopsied fragments are limited to mucosa and part of the submucosa. Furthermore, histologically the differentiation between ischemic colitis and *Clostridium difficile* colitis can be challenging[23] because injuries in ischemic colitis may be associated with an inflammatory pseudomembrane.

The manifestations of ischemic injury of the colon can be patchy, involve the entire large bowel, or have a segmental distribution. No correlation between the length of colonic involvement and the distribution of the superior mesenteric artery and vein and inferior mesenteric artery and vein has been established.[24] The splenic flexure, descending colon, and sigmoid are most commonly involved. The descending and sigmoid colon seem to be the predominant location of colonic ischemia, occurring in about 50% to 75% of patients.[22] The splenic flexure is involved in about 25% to 50% of individuals,[22] whereas rectal ischemia is rare (3%) because of the excellent collateral blood supply of the rectum.[17]

Some causes tend to affect specific areas of the bowel.[10] For example, ischemia secondary to chronic renal failure usually involves the right colon, whereas the most common nonocclusive ischemia involves the junction between the distribution of the superior and inferior mesenteric arteries near the splenic flexure (Griffiths point) and the anastomotic plexus between the inferior mesenteric artery distribution and the hypogastric vascular supply (Sudeck point) at the rectosigmoid junction.[25] Hemorrhagic shock caused by penetrating or blunt trauma predominating in young patients may lead to right-sided ischemic changes.[26] The length of the bowel affected has some correlation with the cause of the ischemia; atheromatous emboli result in short segmented changes, whereas nonocclusive injuries usually involve much longer portions of the colon.

In some cases, other organs, such as the spleen, the kidney, or the gallbladder, may also be involved by the ischemic process (Fig. 1).

CLINICAL FINDINGS

The clinical presentation varies with underlying cause, extent of vascular obstruction, rapidity of ischemic insult, degree of collateral circulation, and presence of comorbidity. Most patients have abdominal pain. The pain is commonly localized to the left lower quadrant because the left colon is most commonly affected. The pain is typically abrupt in onset, crampy, and mild, and frequently accompanied by an urgent desire to defecate. The second key finding is gastrointestinal bleeding, typically mild and not requiring transfusions. Other symptoms include abdominal distension, anorexia, and nausea and vomiting from an associated ileus.

Data on patients hospitalized with a final diagnosis of ischemic colitis are available to represent the frequency of the different clinical findings. The misdiagnosis of numerous cases of transient ischemic injuries may result in underestimation of symptoms associated with this condition. By pooling four recent studies with a combined 515 patients,[2,19,27,28] we found that the most important risk factors were hypertension in 66% of patients, cardiovascular disease in 50% of patients, diabetes mellitus in 29% of patients, chronic renal failure in 22% of patients, and diabetes mellitus in 29% of patients. The mean age of the patients was 70 years and the gender distribution was similar. The two most common clinical findings were abdominal pain encountered in 68% of patients and melena or rectal bleeding found in 54% of patients.

Clinical examination shows mild to moderate tenderness over the involved intestinal segment, abdominal distention, low-grade pyrexia,

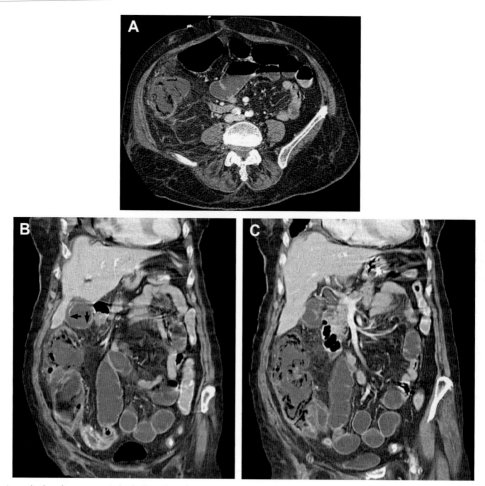

Fig. 1. Association between right ischemic colitis and ischemic cholecystitis. On the axial slice (*A*) and on the coronal reformations (*B, C*), CT shows lack of enhancement and pneumatosis of the right colonic wall. Note also the edema around the gallbladder and the interruption of the gallbladder wall (*arrows*). Surgery and pathology showed ischemia of the right colon and of the gallbladder.

tachycardia, and fecal occult blood. About 10% to 20% have peritoneal signs from colonic necrosis.

The degree of laboratory abnormalities parallels the severity of ischemia. Severe ischemia manifests with leukocytosis with neutrophilia. Necrosis can cause metabolic acidosis and elevations of the serum lactate, phosphate, and alkaline phosphatase levels. These laboratory abnormalities are uncommon with mild ischemia.

ULTRASOUND
Ultrasound Findings

US shows a hypoechoic thickening of the colonic wall. This thickening is circumferential, with bowel wall layers less distinctly differentiated and not always preserved (**Fig. 2**), particularly in transmural forms. The mean bowel thickness ranges from 8 to 11 mm according to the published studies.[29–32] Sudden transition from the normal to the

ischemic segment is frequently seen (**Fig. 3**). The distribution and the length of the bowel thickening are diagnostic points: the distribution is segmental, without discontinuity, and the length of the segment involved is 10 cm or more with a mean affected colon length of 19 cm in the study of Ripolles and colleagues.[29] The colitis involves the left colon in 80% of cases, and is present in the splenic flexure, descending colon, and sigmoid altogether in 50% of cases.[29] Isolated rectal ischemia is exceptional, whereas isolated sigmoid colitis may be encountered in 10% of cases making the differential diagnosis with diverticulitis difficult. The pericolic fat is generally not altered in the nontransmural colitis, whereas altered pericolic fat and absence of improvement in follow-up studies are factors associated with transmural necrosis.[29] At Doppler examination, color flow is absent or barely visible in 80% of cases. Absence of color flow in the bowel wall may be a sign of necrosis,

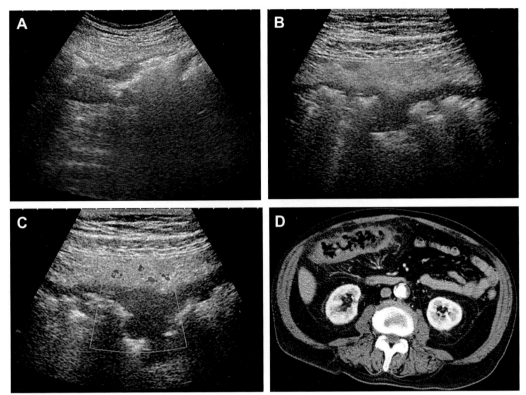

Fig. 2. US appearance of transverse ischemic colitis. US (*A*) shows a circumferential thickening of the bowel wall. On high-resolution examination (*B*) there is no stratification and no flow inside the bowel wall (*C*). Note the fat stranding around the colon, with hyperechoic fat, confirmed by CT (*D*).

whereas the proof of color flow is a good prognostic sign.[31] In contrast to color Doppler, spectral analysis of proximal mesenteric arteries is not helpful because proximal vessels are generally not involved in ischemic colitis and stenosis of mesenteric vessels does not mean ischemia because they are often identified by Doppler in asymptomatic patients older than 65 years.

In summary, an ischemic cause should be suspected in elderly patients presenting with a segmental wall thickening of a long colon segment (>10 cm), particularly on the left side, without any haustration seen and with barely visible or no color Doppler signal intensity.

Ultrasound: Differential Diagnosis

The main differential diagnoses of ischemic colitis on US include neoplasm, inflammation, and infection.[33,34] Most primary neoplasms of the gastrointestinal tract present as short (<10 cm) asymmetric lesions of bowel wall thickening with abrupt margins and no stratification.[33] Diverticulitis generally involves the sigmoid colon with a marked fat infiltration around diverticula, whereas ischemic colitis is rarely localized on the sigmoid colon only. Inflammatory bowel thickening generally preserves stratification, which is inconstant in ischemic colitis. Both inflammation and ischemia, at some stage, cause edema, hemorrhage, inflammation, and ulceration of the bowel, explaining why there is no difference between bowel wall thickness in patients who have inflammation and ischemia.[32] By contrast, color Doppler findings should prompt a strong consideration for ischemia. In the series of Teefey and colleagues,[32] 86% of the cases of ischemic flow were barely visible or not shown with color Doppler flow, compared with 90% of the patients who had acute inflammatory disease who showed abundant color Doppler flow at the wall level. In infectious colitis, most of the cases are limited to the right colon, the longitudinal view of the ascending colon shows the typical haustration pattern (accordion sign) caused by mucosal and submucosal thickening on the one side and by contraction on the other side, lesions are usually confined to the bowel wall, stratification is preserved, and changes of the surrounding structures are absent.[30,34] Color Doppler US shows increased vascularity, which can be used for differentiation from ischemic disease.[32]

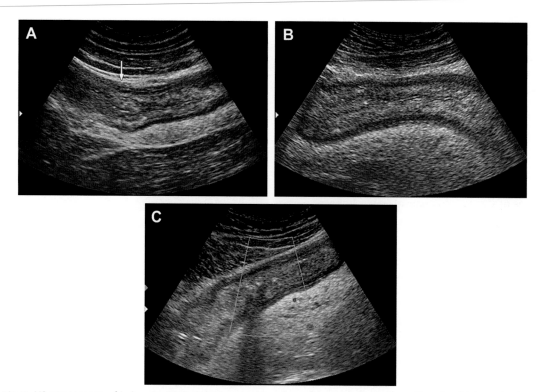

Fig. 3. US appearance of ischemic colitis. (A) The transition from the normal colonic wall to the thickened colonic wall (*arrow*) is clearly seen. (B, C) There is symmetric thickening of the colonic wall with a conservation of the stratification.

Ultrasound Pitfalls

US pitfalls in the diagnosis of ischemic colitis are caused by false negatives and the lack of specificity of bowel thickening that can be observed in several disorders.

False-negative sonographic studies can be explained by several circumstances. In patients who have early ischemia, imaging findings can be normal. Ischemic colitis with wall thinning can be missed on sonography, although this circumstance is more frequent in acute mesenteric ischemia. In the same way, pneumatosis intestinalis, a finding easily shown by CT, is barely seen on US. Also, the sonographic evaluation of the splenic flexure, behind the ribs, and especially of the rectum on transabdominal sonography, may be limited and therefore may be the cause of a false-negative examination.

The most common other causes of colonic wall thickening are neoplasm and infectious or inflammatory processes. The length of the colon involvement (≥ 10 cm) is an argument against tumor. When ischemic colitis is the result of colonic carcinoma, however, it may prove difficult to distinguish between the neoplastic and the ischemic segments on the basis of sonographic findings. For differentiating an ischemic process from an inflammatory process, the absence or the decrease of the color Doppler flow is an argument for ischemia. In the study published by Ripolles,[29] in 20% (n = 9) of the 46 patients in whom bowel wall flow was evaluated, hyperemia of the thickened wall was noted, with readily visible color Doppler flow, all corresponding to patients who had transient ischemia. Ischemic segment hyperemia has already been reported on angiography in some cases of reversible ischemic colitis.[35] It is likely that increased vascularization is shown in such patients because of the realization of imaging during the reperfusion phase. In routine clinical practice, these patients would be indistinguishable from patients who have active inflammatory disease.

CT
CT Findings

Many patients who have inflammatory or infectious types of colitis present with abdominal pain, and multidetector CT is often used as the initial imaging test. As is the case for US, the segmental distribution is a key diagnostic point. In the study by Balthazar and colleagues,[24] a segmental distribution was apparent in 89% of the 54 patients, with the right colon affected in 30%, transverse colon in 9%, left colon in 46%, sigmoid colon in 4%, and the entire colon in 11%. The mean length of involvement in patients who had segmental involvement as detected by CT was 19 cm, and circumferential bowel wall thickness varied greatly from 2 to 20 mm, with a mean thickness of 8 mm.[24] The morphology of the thickening is related to the timing of the examination and to the pathophysiology of the developing anoxic process. In the initial phases of anoxia, mucosal damage occurs first; with more severe and prolonged forms of anoxia, submucosal hemorrhage, edema, and pericolic congestive and edematous changes develop later. Findings may resolve at each of the stages or evolve to infarction. CT appearance is linked to the evolutive phase and may be grouped in three main categories, as shown by Balthazar and colleagues[24] and more recently by Romano and colleagues:[22]

- The wet appearance with a wall thickening with heterogeneous enhancement, showing an acute process. At the initial stage, Romano has described the "little rose" sign (Fig. 4), attributable to hyperdensity of mucosa and to submucosal edema that is more evident at the level of the left colon in the CT axial scan.[36] Acute pathologic changes, particularly after reperfusion of the ischemic bowel, may be responsible for concentric rings (double halo or target sign) with submucosal edema, which becomes evident (Fig. 5). At the acute phase, there is a shaggy contour of the colon and various degrees of pericolic streakiness.
- The dry appearance with concentric and symmetric mild mural thickening and homogeneous attenuation of the wall of the colon

with a sharply defined contour (Fig. 6) and without or with only minimal pericolic streakiness. This finding is the consequence of the progression of the ischemic damage without reperfusion.
- The intramural gas with gas bubbles arranged in a linear fashion (Fig. 7) and best visualized with the window settings for bone or lung.

Even if most ischemic colitis is nonocclusive, CT looks for thrombosis of the mesenteric arteries or veins, or stenosis of mesenteric arteries, although arterial insufficiency is more often responsible for chronic mesenteric ischemia than for colitis. Stenosis or occlusion of at least two of the major vessels is required to establish the diagnosis of arterial insufficiency.

CT: Differential Diagnosis

The differential diagnoses of ischemic colitis on CT depends on the phase and consequently on the appearance of the wall thickening. A stratified thickening suggests infectious colitis, inflammatory colitis, and radiation damage, in which changes are localized to the radiation port, which is commonly the pelvis.[37,38] A homogeneous gray wall thickening (dry form) suggests ulcerative and granulomatous colitis and overall malignancy.[38] Evidence for a benign diagnosis is tapered edges and uniform, symmetric, and thinner thickness. A colonic pneumatosis suggests other causes of pneumatosis, which are numerous, including bowel obstruction and distension, pneumatosis cystoides intestinalis with a cystic pattern of intramural air, inflammatory bowel disease, organ transplantation, obstructive pulmonary diseases, systemic diseases, and instrumental procedures, such as endoscopy or CT colonography.[39]

CT Pitfalls

Despite technical advances that have improved image resolution, there are potential pitfalls in the assessment of the presence and degree of bowel wall thickening in the absence of colonic cleansing or colonic distention in this group of elderly sick patients. Although slight variations (3–4 mm) in the apparent degree of colonic wall thickening can be misleading, marked thickening (>1 cm) is a reliable abnormality when encountered even in partially collapsed segments of bowel. Other potential pitfalls include atypical localization. Isolated right colon involvement is now well known, described in 25% to 30% of ischemic colitis, and is particularly common in shock bowel and in ischemic colitis in patients who have chronic kidney disease, especially when they are on hemodialysis.

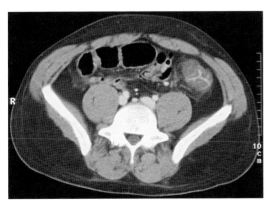

Fig. 4. "Little rose" appearance of the left colon. This finding is due to the hyperdensity of the mucosa.

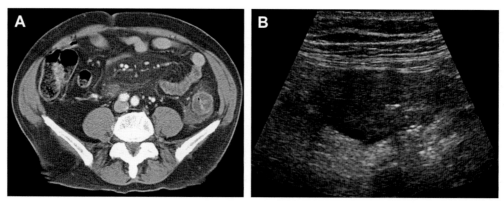

Fig. 5. Wet pattern of ischemic colitis. CT (*A*) shows a target finding with an enhancement of the mucosal and muscular layers and marked fat stranding. This appearance is not specific to ischemia and may be encountered in infections or inflammatory colitis. The disparity of stratification on US (*B*) is an argument for the ischemic origin.

Two rare localizations must be kept in mind: involvement limited to the rectosigmoid (**Fig. 8**),[40] encountered in elderly patients who have atherosclerosis and identified risk factors, and involvement limited to the cecum (**Fig. 9**),[41] because in some cases the cecal arteries may arise directly from either the ileal artery or the colic artery, and consequently the cecum may not benefit from the collateral supply afforded by the vascular arcade.

The interpretation of a pneumatosis is now a now well-reported potential pitfall. Air in the colonic wall is considered a helpful finding of colonic infarction in a proper clinical setting. Numerous other causes of colonic pneumatosis are possible in a patient who has acute abdominal pain,

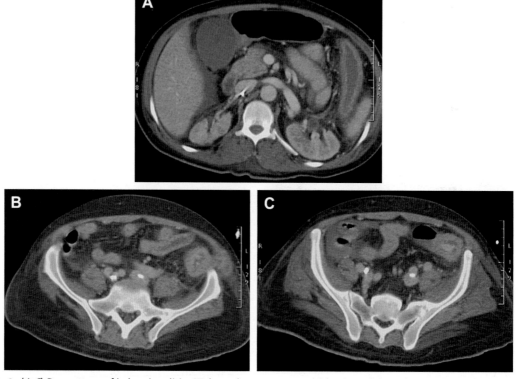

Fig. 6. (*A-C*) Dry pattern of ischemic colitis. CT shows homogeneous thickening of the colon involving the left part of the transverse colon and the left colon.

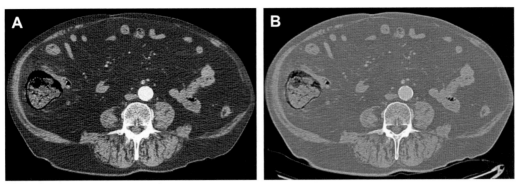

Fig. 7. (*A, B*) Pneumatosis in cecal ischemia. There is a linear cecal pneumatosis clearly shown on both abdominal and lung windows. A cecal resection was performed that confirmed the cecal wall necrosis.

however. The main cause is high-grade intestinal obstruction predominantly attributable to cancer with mural discontinuity. We have shown that in large bowel obstruction, half of the cecal pneumatosis was unrelated to cecal transmural necrosis (**Fig. 10**).[42] Other causes of pneumatosis are listed in the previous paragraph. Evidence of infarction in

colonic pneumatosis is the absence of parietal enhancement.

Distinguishing tumoral from ischemic segments in patients who have ischemic colitis proximal to colonic carcinoma is important to give true evaluation of the length of the tumoral segment and to adapt the surgical procedure. On CT, the ischemic

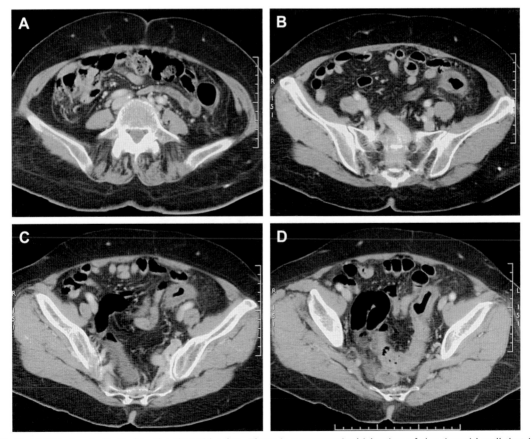

Fig. 8. (*A-D*) Ischemia limited to the sigmoid colon. There is a symmetric thickening of the sigmoid wall that is homogeneously enhanced and without fat stranding, suggestive of a dry pattern. The left colon (*A*) and the rectum (*D*) are normal.

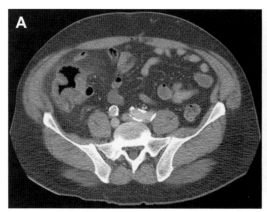 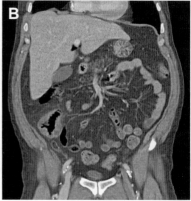

Fig. 9. Ischemia limited to the cecum. Circumferential thickening of the cecal wall seen on axial slice (*A*) and coronal reformation (*B*) in a patient under hemodialysis.

segments are concentrically and smoothly thickened and generally homogeneously enhanced.[43] More atypical is the development of segmental wall thickening in the colonic loop distal to colonic carcinoma in which the distal colon is involved by edema or colitis of nonischemic colitis.[44]

DIAGNOSTIC STRATEGY
Ultrasound or CT?

CT and US are widely used to assess patients who have nonspecific abdominal pain or who are suspected of having colitis.[30,45] Both examinations have advantages compared with endoscopy or barium enema not only in demonstrating the bowel wall but also in outlining the pericolic soft tissues and adjacent structures. The major advantage of CT is the complete demonstration of the abdomen and retroperitoneum free of overlying structures

and the staging of the mesenteric vessels. The radiation dose delivered by CT does not constitute a problem in patients suspected of having ischemic colitis, who are often old. Multiplanar CT allows accurate multiplanar reformations helpful for demonstrating the extent of disease and provides detailed information on complications, such as strictures. Consequently, in clinical practice CT is almost universally accepted as the primary screening modality for the evaluation of patients suspected of having colonic disease. The main finding seen on CT in ischemic colitis is the thickening of the colonic wall. Although this is a nonspecific sign on CT images and can be seen in inflammatory, ischemic, or neoplastic processes, some CT features, such as the amount of wall thickening, extent of disease, enhancement of the colon wall, pericolic reaction, presence of ascites, formation of fistulae, and type of complication

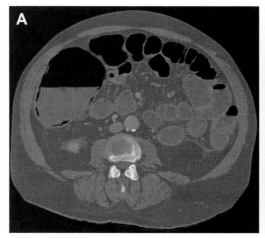 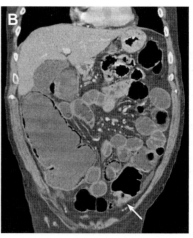

Fig. 10. Pneumatosis consecutive to a large bowel obstruction. Axial slice (*A*) and coronal reformation (*B*) show a cecal pneumatosis with dilatation of the entire right colon. The large bowel dilatation was due to a sigmoid cancer clearly seen (*arrow*) on the coronal view (*B*). At surgery, there was no finding of ischemia on the cecum.

can be used to narrow the differential diagnosis. Comparing US to CT, US provides more detailed information on the different bowel wall layers because of the higher resolution and the better soft tissue contrast. Furthermore, Doppler color allows a semiquantitative assessment of the vascularization of the colonic wall. We consider the use of US for the diagnosis of ischemic colitis as a second-look examination (see **Fig. 5**) after the CT identification of a thickening of the colonic wall if there is doubtful differential diagnosis with tumor or inflammatory process. Ischemic colitis is characterized by greater increases in wall thickness compared with that seen with inflammation, more frequent loss of wall stratification, and absence of flow on color Doppler. By contrast, the thickening is less important, with a more frequent conservation of the stratification, and overall it is symmetric and extended on a greater length when compared with tumor.

ARGUMENTS FOR POSITIVE DIAGNOSIS

Whatever the potential of US and CT to analyze the bowel wall, the positive diagnosis of ischemic colitis is mainly performed by clinical context and the identification of a segmental thickening extended on a significant length, without discontinuity, and without rectal involvement. The analysis of the bowel wall's stratification, enhancement on CT, flow on color Doppler, and significance and symmetry of the thickening gives evidence to differentiate ischemic colitis from other conditions, such as inflammation, infection, or tumor (**Table 1**).

ARGUMENTS FOR SEVERITY DIAGNOSIS

Colonic ischemia remains a disease of variable clinical evaluation and outcome. Two distinct forms of ischemic colitis have been described repeatedly throughout the last 40 years. The spontaneous, usually self-limiting, form of ischemic colitis contrasts drastically with the often catastrophic, more fulminant form. Despite the widely divergent outcomes, the initial presentations of the two forms may be identical.[1–6] Although most patients who have ischemic colitis do survive with conservative therapy, there is a subgroup of patients who require surgery and have a much worse prognosis, particularly if this surgery is delayed. Consequently, it would be important to recognize forms who evoluate through infarction. Clinical and anatomic factors have a prognostic value. There was less hypertension, diabetes mellitus, and rectal bleeding, and more hemodialysis in the patients who had severe

Table 1
Ultrasound and CT diagnostic criteria for differential diagnoses

	Localization	Amount of Thickening (mm)	Extent	Small Bowel Involvement	Rectal Involvement	CT Target Finding	US Stratification	Haustration Conservation	Color Doppler Flow
Ischemia	Left > Right	8–10	Long	+	-	+	+	-	+
Crohn	Right > Left	10–15	Long	+ + +	+	+ +	+ + +	+	+ + +
Ulcerative colitis	Left	6–8	Long	-	+ + +	+ +	+ + +	-	+ + +
Infection	Right > Left	8–10	Long	+ +	+	+ + +	+ + +	+ +	+ + +
Pseudomembranous colitis	Left > Right	10–15	Long	-	-	+ + +	+ + +	+ + +	+ + +
Neoplasia	Predominantly sigmoid	>10	Short	-	-	-	-	-	+ +

colitis compared with the patients who had moderate colitis.[46] Longo and colleagues[47] and Gandhi and colleagues[5] have shown that duration of symptoms, coexisting medical illness, and hypovolemic shock are associated with complicated ischemic colitis requiring surgery. They also noted an increased mortality related to age and to onset of ischemic colitis soon after surgery for an abdominal aneurysm.[47] From a morphologic point of view, patients who had severe ischemic colitis had significantly more right and less left and splenic flexure colonic involvement. The extent of colonic lesions is not in itself associated with a poor outcome. In the same way, the degree of thickening on CT[24] or US, the pattern of a wet edematous or a dry CT appearance,[24] or the conservation of the stratification on US[31] was not correlated with the presence or development of colonic infarction. The prognostic factors useful in clinical practice are the lack of enhancement of the bowel wall (**Fig. 11**) and the presence of intramural gas on CT[24] and the absence of arterial flow in the colonic flow at color Doppler sonography. The large spectrum of disease with pneumatosis has already been evoked, however, and the value of absence of flow initially described has not been confirmed in a more recent study. The absence of flow may be attributable to technical factors (the flow rate being too low to allow detection with currently available sonographic equipment) and to patient-related variables, including overweight patients and breathing motion artifacts in patients who are uncooperative because of serious illness. Moreover, the disappearance of parietal flow in the sonographic follow-up of some patients has been observed, coinciding with clinical improvement in relation to resolution of the ischemic process.[29] Last, flow may be present despite infarction because some toxins released during reperfusion of the ischemic segment can contribute to the pathogenesis of severe intestinal necrosis.[29] Altered pericolic fat (edematous form) was considered as a sign of transmural necrosis on US[29] but not on CT,[24] making this finding questionable for a prognostic use in clinical practice.

In severe forms, ischemic colitis may be perforated with clinical and imaging patterns of gastrointestinal perforation. The goal of imaging is to recognize the site and the cause of perforation (**Fig. 12**).

In summary, US and CT semiology is not accurate to prospectively diagnose patients who need surgery because of the development of infarction. The only proved and useful findings in practice are the presence of intramural gas, of value if associated with the absence of parietal enhancement,[22] or the identification of a colonic wall that remains thin and unenhanced associated with dilatation of the lumen.[45] Because these findings are not constant in patients who will develop colonic infarction, prompt recognition of persistent disease by a close clinical follow-up is essential to successfully manage ischemic colitis. Serial imaging examination, in conjunction with active clinical follow-up, could be an effective method to monitor the course of the ischemic process.

ARGUMENTS FOR CAUSE

Colonic ischemia may be categorized as occlusive or nonocclusive. The most common nonocclusive diseases can be due to low flow states, drugs, or colonic obstruction. Occlusive ischemic colitis may have an arterial or rarely a venous origin. Arterial causes include thrombosis, embolus, injury to the mesenteric vessels during aortic reconstructive surgery, trauma, and small vessel disease caused by diabetes, amyloidosis, radiation injury, or vasculitides. Venous obstruction may be secondary to hypercoagulable states, pancreatitis, portal hypertension, diverticulitis, or trauma.

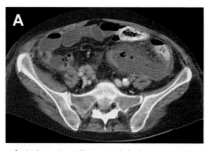
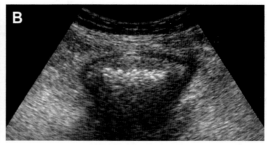

Fig. 11. Left ischemic colitis. CT (*A*) shows a symmetric thickening of the wall of the left colon without any enhancement. On US (*B*), there is some conservation of the stratification with the submucosal layer hyperechoic compared with the muscular layer. Medical management was not sufficient and surgery with colon resection confirmed the diagnosis of ischemic colitis.

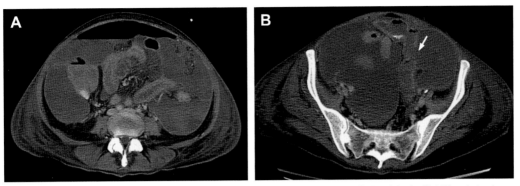

Fig. 12. Sigmoid perforation attributable to ischemic colitis. CT shows fluid and air with air–fluid levels in the peritoneum (*A*). Perforation is located on the left border of the sigmoid colon (*arrow, B*). There is no thickening of the bowel wall and no diverticula are identified. Surgery and pathology confirmed the perforation due to ischemic colitis.

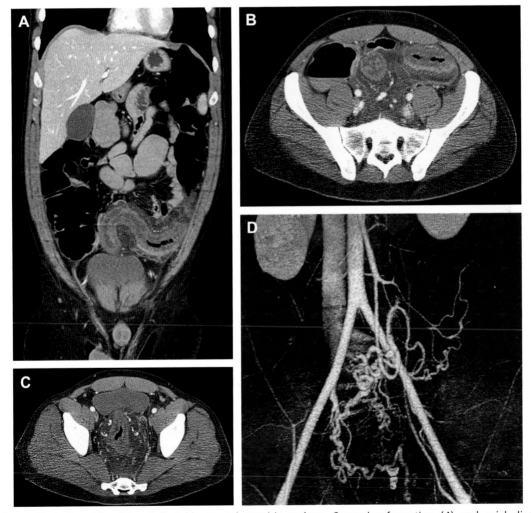

Fig. 13. Rectosigmoid colitis attributable to polyarteritis nodosa. Coronal reformation (*A*) and axial slices (*B, C*) show a thickening of the sigmoid colon with a target finding due to the enhancement of the mucosal and muscular layers. Note the involvement of the upper part of the rectum and the hypervascularization seen on the vascular reformation (*D*). Clinical and CT findings resolved under steroid therapy.

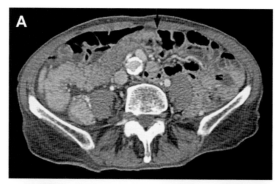

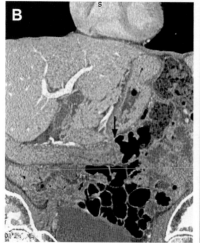
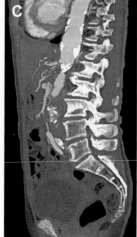
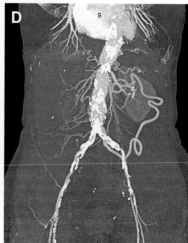

Fig. 14. Ischemic colitis, involving the right colon and the right part of the transverse colon, attributable to splanchnic thromboses. Axial slice (*A*) and curved reformatting (*B*) show thickening of the colon wall with a sudden transition (*arrow*) between the right part of the diseased transverse colon and the left part of the healthy transverse colon. Maximum intensity projection (MIP) sagittal view (*C*) shows thrombosis of the ostia of the celiac trunk and of the superior mesenteric artery. MIP coronal view (*D*) shows the Riolan supply from the inferior mesenteric artery.

Some imaging findings may give evidence for the diagnosis of causes. They are related to the length of the bowel wall involved, to the amount of thickening, and to the direct identification of a vascular obstruction. Regarding the length of the bowel involved, atheromatous emboli result in short segmented changes, whereas nonocclusive injuries usually involve much longer portions of the colon.[48] Regarding the thickness of the bowel wall, it is more pronounced if the bowel ischemia is caused by occlusion of the mesenteric vein than by occlusion of the mesenteric artery alone.[45] When ischemic colitis is attributable to vasculitides, a target sign is more common than a dry appearance,[49] and ischemic lesions relatively commonly involve the rectum (**Fig. 13**) in the same way that in small bowel ischemia due to vasculitides the duodenum is commonly involved.[50] The diagnosis is of importance because patients may be conservatively treated with intravenous high-dose steroid therapy.

Abnormalities of the mesenteric vessels are uncommonly reported in ischemic colitis because the predominant causes are nonocclusive. They have not been individualized in the study of Balthazar[24] with CT performed with 10-mm sections, whereas they have been reported in 10% of cases in the study of Romano[22] with CT performed with 3-mm sections. Care must be given to the splanchnic arteries by looking for stenosis or obstruction attributable to thrombosis (**Fig. 14**) or embolus and to the splanchnic vein by looking for thrombosis or phlebosclerosis.

REFERENCES

1. Huguier M, Barrier A, Boelle PY, et al. Ischemic colitis. Am J Surg 2006;192:679–84.
2. Scharff JR, Longo WE, Vartanian SM, et al. Ischemic colitis: spectrum of disease and outcome. Surgery 2003;134:624–30.

3. Korotinski S, Katz A, Malnick SDH. Chronic ischaemic bowel diseases in the aged—go with the flow. Age Ageing 2005;34:10–6.

4. Boley SJ, Schwartz S, Sternhill V. Reversible vascular occlusion of the colon. Surg Gynecol Obstet 1963;116:53–60.

5. Gandhi SK, Hanson MM, Vernava AM, et al. Ischemic colitis. Dis Colon Rectum 1996;39:88–100.

6. Brandt LJ, boley SJ. Colonic ischemia. Surg Clin North Am 1992;72:203–29.

7. Sreenarasimhaiah J. Diagnosis and management of intestinal ischemic disorders. BMJ 2003;326:1372–6.

8. Newman JR, Cooper MA. Lower gastrointestinal bleeding and ischemic colitis. Can J Gastroenterol 2002;16:597–600.

9. Iwashita A, Yao T, Schlemper RJ, et al. Mesenteric phlebosclerosis: a new disease entity causing ischemic colitis. Dis Colon Rectum 2003;46:209–20.

10. Gandhi SK, Longo WE, Kaminski DL. Ischemic colitis. In: Longo WE, Peterson GJ, Jacobs DL, editors. Intestinal ischemia disorders. Pathophysiology and management. St. Louis (MO): Quality Medical Publishing Inc; 1998. p. 221–41.

11. Kyriakos R, Siewert B, Kato E, et al. CT findings in runner's colitis. Abdom Imaging 2006;31:54–6.

12. Menegaux F, Trésallet C, Kieffer E, et al. Aggressive management of nonocclusive ischemic colitis following aortic reconstruction. Arch Surg 2006;141:678–82.

13. Vassiliou I, Papadakis E, Arkadopoulos N, et al. Gastrointestinal emergencies in cardiac surgery. A retrospective analysis of 3,724 consecutive patients from a single center. Cardiology 2008;111:94–101.

14. Kaminski DL, Herrmann VM. Ischemic colitis. In: Cameron J, editor. Current surgical therapy. 2nd edition. Toronto: BC Decker; 1986. p. 110–4.

15. Brandt LJ, Boley SJ. Ischemic and vascular lesions of the bowel (chap 97). In: Sleisenger MH, Fordtran JS, editors. Gastrointestinal disease: pathophysiology, diagnosis, management. 5th edition. Philadelphia: Saunders; 1993. p. 1940–5.

16. Zimmerman BJ, Granger DN. Reperfusion injury. Surg Clin North Am 1992;72:65–83.

17. Bharucha AE, Tremaine WJ, Johnson CD, et al. Ischemic proctosigmoiditis. Am J Gastroenterol 1996;91:2305–9.

18. Yamazaki T, Shirai Y, Sakai Y, et al. Ischemic stricture of the rectosigmoid colon caused by division of the superior rectal artery below Sudeck's point during sigmoidectomy: report of a case. Surg Today 1997;27:254–6.

19. Flobert C, Cellier C, Berger A. Right colonic involvement is associated with severe forms of ischemic colitis and occurs frequently in patients with chronic renal failure requiring hemodialysis. Am J Gastroenterol 2000;95:195–8.

20. Scowcroft CW, Sanowski RA, Kozarek RA. Colonoscopy in ischemic colitis. Gastrointest Endosc 1981;27:156–61.

21. Zuckerman GR, Prakash C, Merriman RB, et al. The colon single-stripe sign and its relationship to ischemic colitis. Am J Gastroenterol 2003;98:2018–22.

22. Romano S, Romano L, Grassi R. Multidetector row computed tomography findings from ischemia to infarction of the large bowel. Eur J Radiol 2007;61:433–41.

23. Dignan CR, Greenson JK. Can ischemic colitis be differentiated from C difficile colitis in biopsy specimens? Am J Surg Pathol 1998;22:773–4.

24. Balthazar EJ, Yen BC, Gordon RB. Ischemic colitis: CT evaluation of 54 cases. Radiology 1999;211:381–8.

25. Rogers AI, David S. Intestinal blood flow and diseases of vascular impairment. In: Haubrich WS, Schaffner F, Berk JE, editors. Gastroenterology. 5th edition. Philadelphia: Saunders; 1995. p. 1212–34.

26. Ludwing K, Quebbeman EJ, Bergstein JM, et al. Shock-associated right colon ischemia and necrosis. J Trauma 1995;39:1171–4.

27. Medina C, Vilaseca J, Videla S, et al. Outcome of patients with ischemic colitis: review of 53 cases. Dis Colon Rectum 2004;47:180–4.

28. Sotiriadis J, Brandt LJ, Behin DS, et al. Ischemic colitis has a worse prognosis when isolated to the right side of the colon. Am J Gastroenterol 2007;102:2247–52.

29. Ripolles T, Simo L, Martinez-Pérez MJ, et al. Sonographic findings in ischemic colitis in 58 patients. AJR Am J Roentgenol 2005;184:777–85.

30. Hollerweger A. Colonic diseases: the value of US examination. EJR 2007;64:239–49.

31. Danse EM, Van Beers BE, Jamart J, et al. Prognosis of ischemic colitis: comparison of color Doppler sonography with early clinical and laboratory findings. AJR 2000;175:1151–4.

32. Teefey SA, Roarke MC, Brink JA. Bowel wall thickening: differentiation of inflammation from ischemia with color Doppler and duplex US. Radiology 1996;198:547–51.

33. Truong M, Atri M, Bret PM, et al. Sonographic appearance of benign and malignant conditions of the colon. AJR 1998;170:1451–5.

34. Danse EM, Jamart J, Hoang P, et al. Focal bowel wall changes detected with colour Doppler ultrasound: diagnostic value in acute non-diverticular diseases of the colon. Br J Radiol 2004;77:917–21.

35. Reuter SR, Kanter IE, Redman HC. Angiography in reversible colonic ischemia. Radiology 1970;97:371–5.

36. Romano S, Lassandro F, Scaglione M, et al. Ischemia and infarction of the small bowel and colon: spectrum of imaging findings. Abdom Imaging 2006;31:277–92.

37. Macari M, Balthazar EJ. CT of bowel wall thickening: significance and pitfalls of interpretation. AJR 2001; 176:1105–15.

38. Wittenberg J, Harisinghani MG, Jhaveri K, et al. Algorithmic approach to CT diagnosis of the abnormal bowel wall. Radiographics 2002;22: 1093–109.

39. Ho LM, Paulson EK, Thompson WM. Pneumatosis intestinalis in the adult: benign to life-threatening causes. AJR 2007;188:1604–13.

40. Sharif S, Hyser M. Ischemic proctitis: case series and literature review. Am Surg 2006;72:1241–7.

41. Mancuso MA, Cheung YY, Silas AM, et al. Case 120: ischemic colitis limited to the cecum. Radiology 2007;244:919–22.

42. Taourel P, Garibaldi F, Arrigoni J, et al. Cecal pneumatosis in patients with obstructive colon cancer: correlation of CT findings with bowel viability. AJR 2004;183:1667–71.

43. Ko GY, Ha HK, Lee HJ, et al. Usefulness of CT in patients with ischemic colitis proximal to colonic cancer. AJR 1997;168:951–6.

44. Jang HJ, Lim HK, Park CK, et al. Segmental wall thickening in the colonic loop distal to colonic carcinoma at CT: importance and histopathologic correlation. Radiology 2000;216:712–7.

45. Thoeni RF, Cello JP. CT imaging of colitis. Radiology 2006;240:623–38.

46. Park CJ, Jang MK, Shin WG, et al. Can we predict the development of ischemic colitis among patients with lower abdominal pain? Dis Colon Rectum 2007; 50:232–8.

47. Longo WE, Ballantyne GH, Gusberg RJ. Ischemic colitis: patterns and prognosis. Dis Colon Rectum 1992;35:726–30.

48. Kaleya RN, Bodey SJ. Colonic ischemia. Perspect Colon Rectal Surg 1990;3:62–81.

49. Byun JY, Ha HK, Yu SY, et al. CT features of systemic lupus erythematosus in patients with acute abdominal pain: emphasis on ischemic bowel disease. Radiology 1999;211:203–19.

50. Kim JK, Ha HK, Byun JY, et al. CT differentiation of mesenteric ischemia due to vasculitis and thromboembolic disease.

Ischemia and Infarction of the Intestine Related to Obstruction

Stefania Romano, MD[a],*, Giovanni Bartone, MD[b],
Luigia Romano, MD[a]

KEYWORDS

- Bowel obstruction • Ischemia • Infarction
- MDCT • Acute abdomen

The term "intestinal obstruction" indicates various conditions that, although unlike in character, have the common property of mechanically presenting an obstacle to transit along the intestine.[1] The obstructing agent may be different: peritoneal adhesions (**Figs. 1** and **2**), neoplasm, torsion of a loop around an axis (**Fig. 3**), invagination of a certain portion of the bowel into the segment below (**Fig. 4**), presence of obstructing gross endoluminal material, inflammatory stenosis, and internal or external hernias. Patients with intestinal obstruction may present with acute or chronic conditions, mainly depending on the underlying cause of occlusion and the intestinal segment involved.

Traditionally, classification of the degree of obstruction defined "occlusion" as complete closure of the intestinal lumen with impossible passage of contents (eg, strangulation and torsion) and "obstruction" as incomplete closure of the lumen with difficult passage of contents (eg, invagination, obturation, stenosis).[1] Since the last century, the significance of early diagnosis has been well known and discussed in every reported series of intestinal obstructions in which reference was made to mortality.[2]

Symptomatology of bowel obstruction is typically represented by pain, vomiting, distension, and constipation. The pain is crampiform and intermittent, whereas distension is present almost invariably when a patient presents to the emergency department.[2] As distinguished from other acute abdominal lesions, vomiting from obstruction tends to be more frequent and abundant and is caused by mechanical block in the bowel that brings a regurgitation of the stagnant endoluminal continent into the higher reaches of the alimentary canal.[2] It is possible to clinically observe instances of mechanical obstructions in which no vomiting occurs despite the conspicuous distension of the bowel; however, these cases are usually found with obstruction of the colon.[2] Whereas chronic obstructions may last for weeks or months, acute obstructions may represent expression of severe disease that is potentially lethal if not recognized early. Although simple mechanical obstruction frequently may be relieved by suction without to the need for immediate operation, complicated obstructions and late-stage occlusions may require true emergency surgery.

PATHOLOGIC CHANGES IN SMALL BOWEL AND COLON

Regarding the general pathology of the bowel occlusions, at the time of the acute occluding accident the involved intestine is normal.[3], Because of its mobility, smooth surface, and relatively small girth, the small intestine seems to be much more likely to be snared by a band than a colon segment.[3] The wall of the small intestine is thinner and frailer, and the effect of strangulation manifests sooner.[3] The colon has stouter walls, sacculi,

[a] Department of Diagnostic Imaging, Section of General and Emergency Radiology, "A. Cardarelli" Hospital, Naples, Italy
[b] Emergency Surgery, "A. Cardarelli" Hospital, Naples, Italy
* Corresponding author. Via Giuseppe Fava 28 parco la piramide, 80016 Marano di Napoli (NA), Italy.
E-mail address: stefromano@libero.it (S. Romano).

Radiol Clin N Am 46 (2008) 925–942
doi:10.1016/j.rcl.2008.07.004

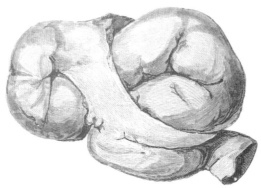

Fig. 1. Strangulation by a broad peritoneal band passing between two adjacent segments of ileum. (*From* Treves F. Intestinal obstruction. New York: William Wood & Co; 1899. p. 30.)

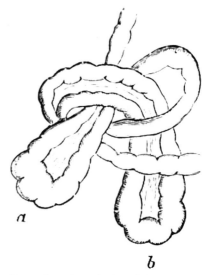

Fig. 3. Illustration of a volvulus of the small intestine. (*From* Treves F. Intestinal obstruction. New York: William Wood & Co; 1899. p. 140.)

and appendices epiploicae, which may offer obstacles to the smooth gliding of a loop beneath a band. If lightly snared, the disposition of its muscular layers would facilitate its escape.[3] The nerve supply of the small bowel is elaborate, whereas the nervous organization of the large bowel is poorer; its connections with the great nerve centers of the abdomen are less intimate and direct, as in the case of the jejunum and ileum.[3]

The phenomenon of strangulation is more pronounced if the small intestine is involved than if the snared segment belongs to the colon.[3] If strangulation of the colon produces manifestations equal with those that attend the small bowel, a greater extent of intestine should be involved,[3]

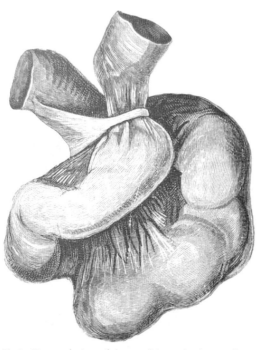

Fig. 2. Strangulation of the small intestine by a solitary band attached at either end to the mesentery. (*From* Treves F. Intestinal obstruction. New York: William Wood & Co; 1899. p. 34.)

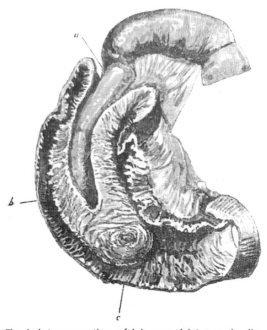

Fig. 4. Intussusception of jejunum. (a) Internal cylinder. (b) Middle cylinder. (c) External cylinder. (*From* Treves F. Intestinal obstruction. New York: William Wood & Co; 1899. p. 142.)

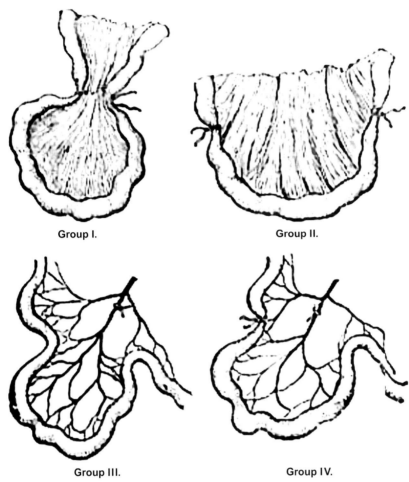

Group I.   Group II.

Group III.   Group IV.

Fig. 5. Illustration of Kader's experiments. (*From* Treves F. Intestinal obstruction. New York: William Wood & Co; 1899. p. 14.)

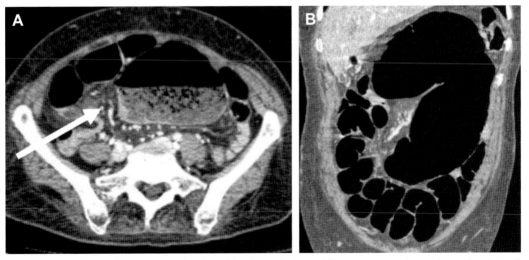

Fig. 6. MDCT scan shows the presence of a sigmoid colon volvulus, with mesentery and vascular peduncle torsion (*A, arrow*) and the closed loop of large bowel, predominantly overdistended by gas, with thin wall and markedly reduced parietal enhancement (*B*). Surgery confirmed the ischemic changes of the involved sigmoid segment.

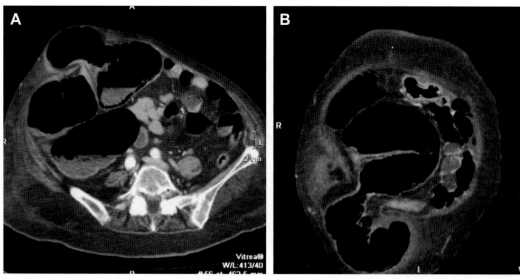

Fig. 7. MDCT finding of strangulated external hernia of the right colon, axial scan (A) and coronal reformatted image (B). There was absence of parietal enhancement and evidence of pneumatosis of the involved closed loop.

as in the sigmoid volvulus. In such instances, what the colon lacks in fineness and sensitivity of structure, it makes up for in the extent of tissue involved.[3] In describing the effects of strangulation, the bowel above the obstruction grows red, the bowel below it grows white, and the coil involved grows livid and purple.[3]

The intestine above the seat of strangulation is distended and filled with gas or fluid; the degree of distension varies, but the bowel may be found to be two or three times its normal size.[3] The distended intestine is a dull red, the tint to a certain degree of congestion. On the serous surface the dilated vessels form a dense tracery.[3] Dilated intestine may be thickened by edema, but no hypertrophy is found. In the absence of edema, the intestinal wall may be thin and pale; this latter condition can be observed in segments that are located at some distance from the obstruction but have taken part in the general distension.[3] The intestinal mucosa close to the obstruction appears swollen, has edema, and is deep red. In the segment just above the obstruction it is not unusual to find superficial erosions (not ulcers, which are most common to the intestine above a stenosis).[3]

Gangrenous patches can be found in the wall of the intestine that lies immediately above the involved loop, particularly in cases of long-standing strangulated obstructions.[3] The intestine below the obstruction is pale, contracted, and empty; however, a definite degree of congestion can be noted.[3] The late-stage obstructed loop appears congested and edematous. As the engorgement increases, the color changes from dark blue to

reddish blue, to port wine color, and finally to black.[3] The snared bowel preserves its normal smooth and lustrous surface for a while, but it is soon replaced by a dull, cloudy, sticky appearance.[3] The necrotic intestine may present a mere patch of gangrene to destruction of a long intestinal segment; in this dramatic case, perforation occurs.[3]

A crucial point involving intestinal obstructions is the predictability about living or dead bowel. Some studies have shown the pattern of the histopathologic changes of the bowel during different grades of occlusion. In one study by Kader dated 1891, he considered four groups of dogs (**Fig. 5**).[3] In the first group, a loop of intestine was strangulated together with its mesentery, which simulated acute strangulation by a band.[3] When the strangulating cord was not too tightly drawn, the intestinal loop presented first as venous hyperemia and then venous stasis. The wall became edematous and presented with extravasation of blood, with serous exudation in the bowel lumen.[3] When the strangulating cord was drawn as tightly as possible, the loop became pale and then cyanotic. When the blood supply was abruptly and entirely cut off, there was little or no edema, no extravasation, and no exudation into the lumen of the bowel.[3] In any case, the coil of strangulated bowel soon became paralyzed, gas developed, and distension developed.[3] If the loop was apparently empty, gas developed, but if the intestine contained fecal material, the gas formation was more copious.[3] The vessels of the strangulated mesentery became thrombosed and the bowel became necrotic

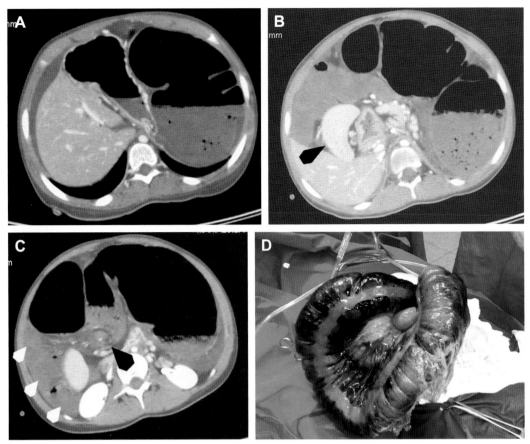

Fig. 8. MDCT finding of intestinal occlusion with infarction in patient with colonic volvolus from mesentery malrotation. Massive distension of the colon (*A–C*), predominantly by air, with complete absence of wall enhancement. Note the wandering spleen (*B, arrowhead*) and the whirl sign from mesenteric torsion (*C, black arrowhead*). The small bowel appears with marked decreased parietal enhancement and wall thickening (*C, white arrowhead*). Surgery confirmed the presence of massive infarction of the large bowel (*D*). The small bowel was ischemic but not necrotic.

in whole or in part, with perforation in a large, solitary hole or in multiple, minute capillary perforations.[3] The bowel above and below the strangulated coil first contracted for a few moments and then became distended, more slowly than in the loop involved in strangulation.[3] The bowel became less contractile but not paralyzed, with congested mucosa and endoluminal stasis.[3] The intestine below the strangulated loop appeared empty and contracted for some extent.[3]

In the second group, an intestinal loop was occluded at two points a short distance from one another, which simulated the conditions surrounding strictures and luminal occlusion by foreign bodies.[3] If the isolated loop contained no intestinal material, a small amount of gas developed; if the intestine contained some material, some gas was formed but in a small amount, which did not lead to bowel distension.[3] Contractility of the intestine

seemed not to be greatly diminished, with no gross changes in the bowel tissue. The intestine above the isolated group became more distended than the involved loop itself and the contractility was slightly reduced, whereas the bowel below remained unchanged or somewhat contracted.[3]

In the third group of Kader's experiment, the bowel was left untouched but the mesentery of a certain loop was ligatured so that the vascular circulation was arrested and the intestinal lumen was free, which simulated conditions of mesenteric vessels thrombosis.[3] In this condition, marked changes took place in the intestinal segment deprived of blood: contractility diminished to paralysis, the wall became thickened and edematous, and exudation took place into the bowel lumen.[3] Much gas developed in the affected segment, and in time the bowel showed the necrosis phenomenon.[3]

Table 1
Schematic spectrum of disease progression in the small bowel obstruction

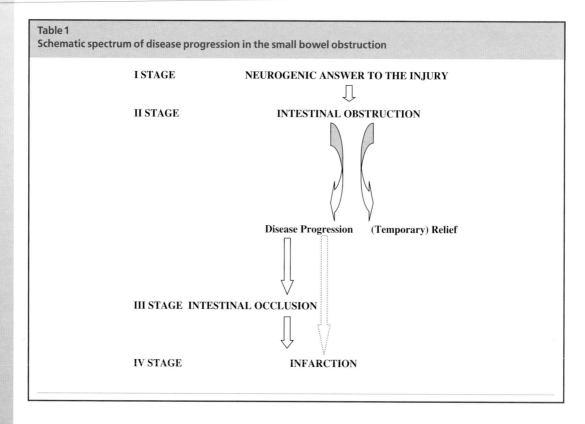

In the last group, the mesentery of a certain loop of intestine was ligatured as in the third group; the bowel immediately above the loop that was deprived of blood was occluded so that no endoluminal matter passing from above could enter the section of intestine attached to the damaged mesentery.[3] The observed changes were similar to those of third group, but the damaged bowel became the seat of local gas distension, despite the fact that nothing could enter it from above and it could be empty below. The intestine above the occlusion became less or more distended.[3] Additional experiments by Scott and Wangensteen indicated that the blood loss factor was significant in strangulating types of obstruction, particularly where the venous obstruction factor predominated.[4]

Blood pressure tracings were made on several dogs after the following procedures: ligature of the veins to a segment of gut, ligature of the arterial supply to a similar segment, complete division of the mesentery of the gut cutting both arteries and veins, and encirclement ligature of a segment of gut and its mesentery.[4] The results of these experiments indicated a direct correlation among the manner of interference with the blood supply of the gut, the arterial blood pressure, and the length of the segment concerned, especially in venous obstructions and the survival time.[4]

The ligation of veins to a segment of small intestine, which varied in length from 2 to 5 feet, caused severe falls in arterial blood pressure that had fatal results in 2 to 4 hours.[4] In one case, in which the superior mesenteric vein was tied, arterial pressure fell gradually, and in 1 hour the dog was dead.[4] Researchers also observed that the longer the loop, the more marked the fall in pressure and

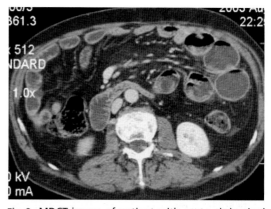

Fig. 9. MDCT image of patient with acute abdominal pain, moderate distension of the small intestine, especially of the loops located at the left quadrant; normal appearance of the wall thickness and enhancement. The patient underwent laparoscopy, lower jejunual adhesions were found.

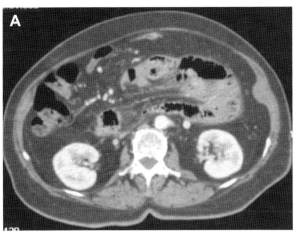
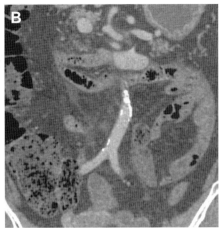

Fig. 10. MDCT scan (A) shows moderate air and fluid distension of some small intestinal loops sited in middle/left abdominal quadrant, which appear normal in parietal thickening and enhancement. Note the moderate edema and engorgement of the mesentery. In the absence of mechanical ileus findings, the coronal reformatted image (B) better shows an anomalous location of the small bowel, which suggests left paraduodenal internal hernia (confirmed at surgery).

the shorter the survival period.[4] The results in the second group, in which the arteries were tied, and in group three were approximately the same[4]: blood pressure tracings that continued for 4 to 6 hours showed no significant alterations in pressure, with a survival time of 16 to 20 hours.[4] In the fourth group, no significant falls in pressure occurred.[4]

From these experiments, researchers noted that the blood loss factor was significant in determining whether an early severe fall in arterial blood pressure would occur. Whether just the arteries or the arteries and veins together were tied did not seem to make a significant difference; however, when the veins alone were tied, a gradual but definite and lethal fall in pressure invariably occurred.[4] As a consequence, it could be determined that increased intraluminal pressure, in instances in which it became great enough to occlude the vein, and the various type of torsion, encirclement, and invagination of the intestine represent conditions of venous obstructions of varying grade.[4]

The primary effects of the obstruction seem to be mechanical and concerning intraenteric pressure as related to absorption, viability, and permeability of the bowel.[5] Within certain limits, however, the bowel wall is able to maintain an adequate blood supply through the process of stretching of its muscular layer.[5] Histologic studies of intestinal occlusions made upon bowel wall in the viable segments showed thinning of the wall and prominent blood vessels exhibiting collections of red cells. There was no interstitial hemorrhage; edema, shortening, and clubbing of the villi

represented consistent findings.[5] In the nonviable segments, interstitial hemorrhage and erosion of the mucosa were common findings.[5] Some factors have been described as local end effects attending sustained worsening of a simple obstruction of a long loop, including increase in intraluminal content (gas and fluid), distension and intestinal stasis, thinning of the intestinal wall, decreased absorption from the intestinal lumen, venous stasis in the bowel wall, anoxemia, clusters of intense myoelectric activity arising and migrating aborally to interrupt quiescent periods of little or no activity, impaired viability, histologic injury to the intestinal wall, and altered permeability.[5,6]

Another crucial point to consider is the presence of strangulating obstruction with little or no evidence of distension. In a usual strangulating obstruction, there are two coexisting varieties of factors, such as the strangulation of a torsioned loop and simple obstruction in the intestine proximal to the site of strangulation.[5] To initiate the strangulating effects of a compromised blood supply in the imprisoned loop, the strangulating mechanism should obstruct the proximal bowel.[5] There could be evidence of strangulating obstruction and a devitalized bowel requiring resection with little or no evidence of distension, however. The lesson to be learned from this is that the return of venous blood from an imprisoned loop of bowel may be impeded without the presence of a mechanical block to the continuity of the intestine.[5]

In obstruction of the colon, the ileocecal valve and sphincter influence its effects and the character of the symptoms. The contents of the upper

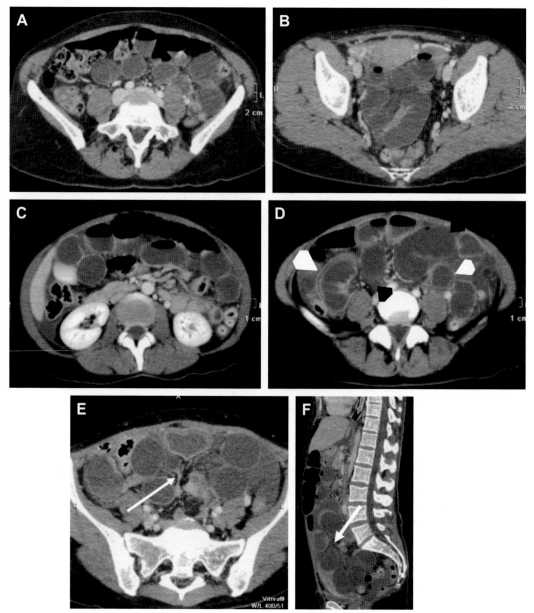

Fig. 11. In this patient with moderate abdominal pain and history of several subocclusive episodes for weeks, MDCT scans showed findings of obstruction to the intestinal transit, with presence of fluid distension of the small intestine (II stage) (*A, B*). She was scheduled for a laparoscopy by the referring surgeon; 2 days after the CT scanning, she experienced acute abdominal pain. MDCT examination showed the findings of a more advanced obstructive disease (III stage) with presence of moderate peritoneal fluid and overdistended fluid filling the small intestine (*C*). Several segments contained parietal thickening characterized by submucosal edema and moderately decreased enhancement (*D, white arrowheads*). Note that some loops appeared with thin walls and decreased enhancement (*D, black arrowhead*). There was also evidence in the pelvis of mesenteric engorgement with converging "vortex" appearance and a band-like structure (*E, F, arrows*). Surgery confirmed the presence of small bowel occlusion from adhesions with ischemia of some segments, which recovered after de-banding. No resection was required.

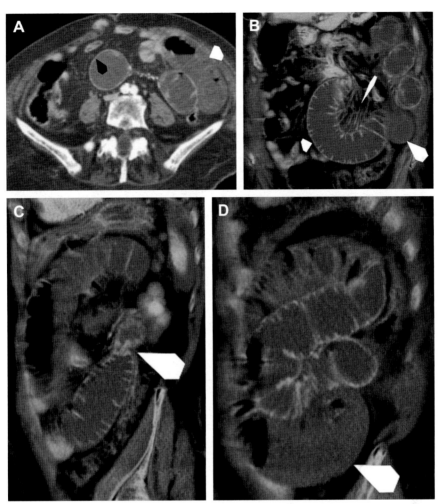

Fig. 12. MDCT images of patient with small bowel volvulus with necrotic loop (IV stage of disease). (*A*) Different appearance of the small intestine segments was appreciable: thin bowel loop with appreciable parietal enhancement (*black arrowhead*) and a thickened segment with absence of enhancement (*white arrowhead*). (*B*) Different pattern of appearance and enhancement are appreciable in the MPR coronal reformatted image: a thin wall dilated segment in which valvulae conniventes are appreciable and not thickened (*small arrowhead*); the thickened and unenhanced segment (*large arrowhead*); and the mesenterial converging engorgement (*thin arrowhead*). (*C*) Multiplanar reformations may allow visualization of the point of the torsion of the loop (*arrowhead*) and a better evaluation of the necrotic segment extension (*D*) (*arrowhead*). Note the collapsed small intestine below the occluded loops by volvulus and the residual feces and air in the colon (*A*).

reaches of the gastrointestinal canal are permitted free entry to the colon, but because of the check-valve nature of the ileocecal juncture, regurgitation from the distended large bowel into the terminal reaches of the small intestine does not occur frequently.[5] In colonic obstructions, distension with development of high intraluminal pressures is common.[5] Sustained pressures in the bowel lumen in excess of capillary pressure are rarely tolerated by the gut wall.[5] In acute conditions, colonic obstruction becomes virtually a short, closed loop occlusion, in which perforation is not a rare occurrence.[5]

Regarding the general pathology of the bowel obstructions, conditions under this heading could be considered bowel strictures or any stenosis of gradual formation.[3] The lumen is narrowed but not occluded, and the intestinal contents can pass, but with difficulty. There is obstruction, but not occlusion[3] Assuming that the narrowing has formed slowly and gradually and there is no acuteness but chronicity, a typical example of this condition involves malignant strictures of the colon.[3] In this case, the bowel below the obstruction is empty and contracted, has a pale color, and has unchanged walls, whereas the colon above the

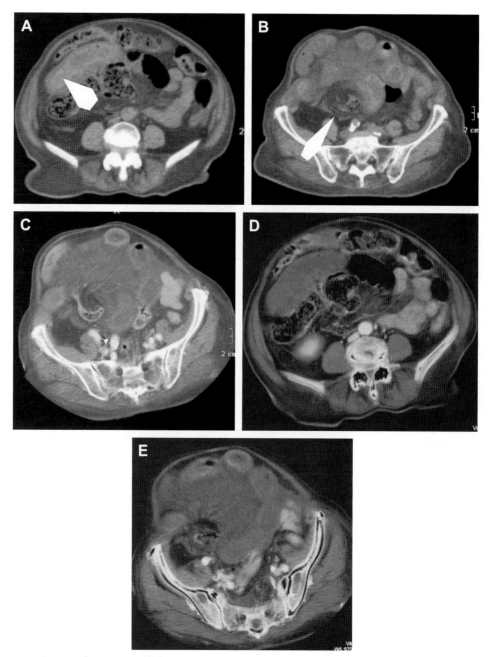

Fig. 13. MDCT images of small bowel infarction from volvulus (IV stage disease). (A) On the unenhanced scans, it is possible to differentiate the spontaneous hyperdensity of the wall and content of a small intestine dilated segment (*arrowhead*) from hemorrhage. (B) A complete 360° whirl sign is also appreciable (*arrowhead*). (C, D) Contrast-enhanced scans confirmed the evidence of a small bowel volvulus with necrosis of the strangulated loops. Note the presence of different stages of disease (normal enhancing, hyperaemic, ischemic, necrotic) in the same patient (A–E).

obstruction becomes dilated (distension may be of high degree) and has hypertrophic walls.[3] This type represents a true hypertrophy of muscle, not a mere hyperplasia, because of the efforts on the part of the intestine to force the endoluminal

material through the narrow tract of the colon.[3] These changes are more intense closer to the stricture.[3] The bowel wall becomes thickened and has prominent vessels. Mucosal thickening and ulcerations suggest inflammatory changes

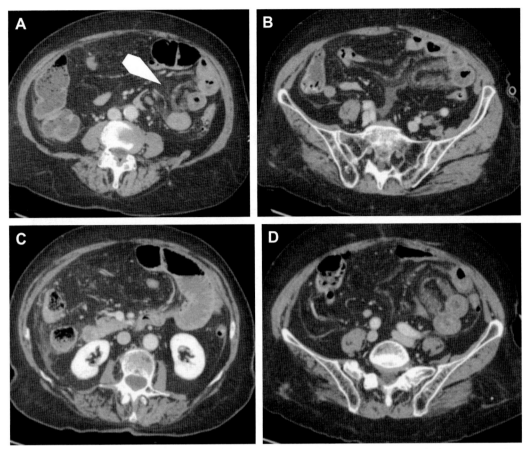

Fig. 14. MDCT of patient with acute abdominal pain and no obstructive symptoms. (A, B) There was no sign of mechanical ileus but evidence of some small bowel loops at the left quadrant characterized by parietal thickening with submucosal edema and hyperdensity of the mucosa, with mesenteric engorgement and fluid. (A) These findings suggest reperfusion injury. Note that an anomalous appearance of the mesentery could be also appreciated (arrowhead), but a first diagnosis of a specific intestinal "flogosis" was made. Symptoms of the patient worsened, and 30 hours later he was referred for a follow-up CT scan: the images showed the presence of increased fluid dilation of the loops located above the thickened small bowel segments (C), which appeared characterized by an increased mucosal hyperdensity and submucosal edema (D). Whirl sign appeared also much evident (C, D; multimedia component*). Note the increased amount of peritoneal fluid. Diagnosis of small bowel obstruction from volvulus was made and confirmed by surgery.

that could be severe, developing complications (eg, perforations, sacculated abscesses, and fistulae), with gangrene developing as a late and dramatic event.[3]

DIAGNOSTIC IMAGING IN ISCHEMIA AND INFARCTION FROM INTESTINAL OBSTRUCTION

Because infarction complications from intestinal obstruction are severe and potentially lethal, the objective of the diagnostic imaging should be early recognition of ischemic findings. (multimedia component 1*).

Large Bowel Obstruction

Because of the different reaction mechanism of the colon to an endoluminal obstacle to the transit, with different timing of obstruction development and symptoms regarding small bowel occlusions, as discussed in the section on general pathology, diagnosis of the large bowel occlusion could be suggested by abdominal radiography and then

---

* Video for this article can be accessed by visiting www.radiologic.theclinics.com. In the online table of contents for this issue, click on "add-ons."

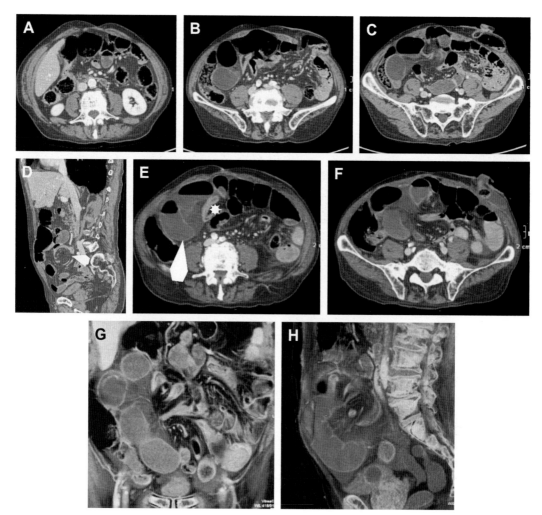

Fig. 15. MDCT findings of patient with left colostomy for previous resection for distal descending colon cancer who had referred abdominal pain for several hours but no definite obstructive symptoms. A first diagnosis of difficult intestinal transit was made from the CT. The appearance of the intestine was not homogeneous: some loops appeared scarcely distended by fluid with endoluminal heterogeneous content, and the remnant colon presented air and feces in the lumen (*A–C*). Some important findings not considered in the report could be useful for a correct diagnosis, however, such as the presence of a thin-walled more dilated loop at the right quadrant (*B*), evidence of mesenteric edema (*C*), and an appreciable whirl sign (*C, D*). The patient's obstructive conditions worsened and 3 days later he underwent a follow-up CT examination because of the acute pain. (*E*) From the MDCT, findings of intestinal advanced ischemia from small bowel volvulus were evident: thin-walled bowel loop with marked decreased parietal enhancement (*arrowhead*) and hyperemic collapsed proximal loop (*asterisk*). (*F–H*) Whirl sign from a closed loop obstruction was evident, which suggested diagnosis of volvulus of the small bowel and late-stage ischemic complication, which were confirmed at surgery.

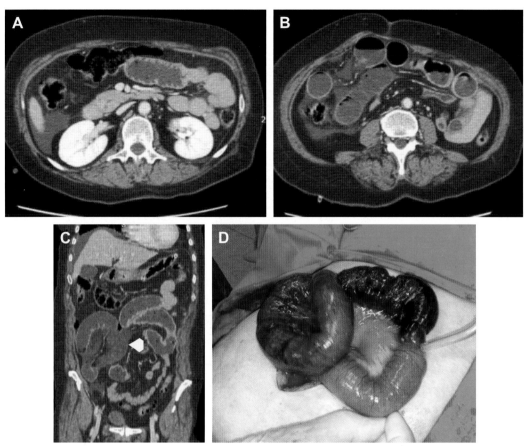

Fig. 16. MDCT of patient with acute abdominal pain and suspicion of small bowel obstruction. (*A, B*) There was evidence of peritoneal fluid and proximal jejunum collapse and fluid distension in the ileum. (*C*) Some segments of dilated intestine showed thin unenhancing wall (*arrowhead*). (*D*) Surgery confirmed the presence of closed loop from adhesions with segmental infarction.

evaluated with CT, which represents an optimal comprehensive imaging method,[7–16] although published data are more limited than data correlated to small intestine obstructions.[15] In emergency situations, most cases of large bowel obstructions that are referred for CT examination are related to late-stage obstruction or strangulated hernia or volvulus (**Figs. 6** and **7**). The evaluation of large bowel ischemia from intestinal obstruction should consider the feature and disposition of the different segments of the large intestine, the evidence of bowel distension by air or fluid, the caliber of the cecum, the parietal thickening of thinning, the presence of the parietal enhancement, the evidence of pneumatosis or pneumoperitoneum, and the presumable cause of the obstruction.

In a study by Taourel and colleagues[15] in 2004, necrosis of the cecum in patients with large bowel occlusion from neoplasm was correlated to CT evidence of thickening of bowel wall, right mesocolic edema, pneumoperitoneum,

cecal pneumatosis, and dilation. The presence of cecal pneumatosis was found in four of six patients with necrosis of the cecum, five patients with right mesocolic edema and pneumoperitoneum, two patients with cecal mural thickening, three patients with dilation of 8 to 12 cm, and one patient with dilation of more than 12 cm.[15] Parietal pneumatosis has been considered a finding correlated to necrosis; however, it can be the result of mucosal disruption caused by colonic overdistension.[15] This study indicated that the high degree of dilation and development of ischemia in a colon segment not close to the tumoral site could be explained by Laplace's law, which states that tension in the bowel wall increases with increased intraluminal pressure and the diameter of the obstructed bowel.[15] In this condition, the mucosal blood flow diminishes, and mucosal or transmural necrosis develops.[15] It is important to differentiate necrotic from viable intestine to plan correct therapeutic management of a patient. CT findings of

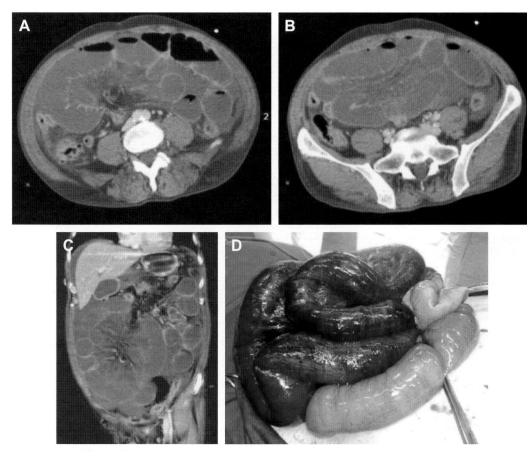

Fig. 17. MDCT findings of late-stage small bowel occlusion. (A) Overdistension of the small intestine with whirl sign evidence and mesenteric engorgement can be appreciated. (B, C) Note the presence of different appearance of the bowel. Some distended loops presented with parietal enhancement, whereas in others the enhancement was appreciable but decreased or markedly reduced or absent. No sign of parietal thickening was noted. (D) Surgery confirmed the intestinal infarction from volvulus of the small intestine and viability of others distended loops not involved in the torsion.

pneumatosis do not always indicate presence of necrosis in patients with intestinal ischemia.[15–18] The study by Taourel and colleagues concluded that cecal pneumatosis in patients with large bowel obstruction from neoplasm may be related to a viable intestine when it displays a bubble-like (more than band-like) appearance or when it is not associated with other findings of ischemia.[15]

Diagnosis of a closed loop obstruction from volvulus of the colon represents an emergency condition in which a prompt radiologic diagnosis is important for patient management. At MDCT, visualization of the whirl sign, which results from twisting of the bowel and branching of the mesenteric vessels, could be increased with the multiplanar reformatting process.[19–20] In the evaluation of MDCT images in a patient with colonic volvulus, it is important to report the status of the distended bowel, whether there is parietal enhancement, and

the presence and location of the beak and whirl. Progressive pathologic changes of the wall from ischemia could reflect those signs related to impaired venous drainage. If difference in timing and appearance can be noted, it is important to note the status of the colonic wall in the segments adjacent to the closed loop to provide important information to the surgeon regarding the surgical intervention required (Fig. 8).

Small Bowel Obstruction

Much information has been provided in scientific literature on acute small bowel obstruction, which is a common clinical condition often associated with signs and symptoms similar to those seen in other acute abdominal disorders. It represents a challenging entity to diagnose.[20] Abdominal radiography seems to represent the first imaging method for symptomatic patients in detection of

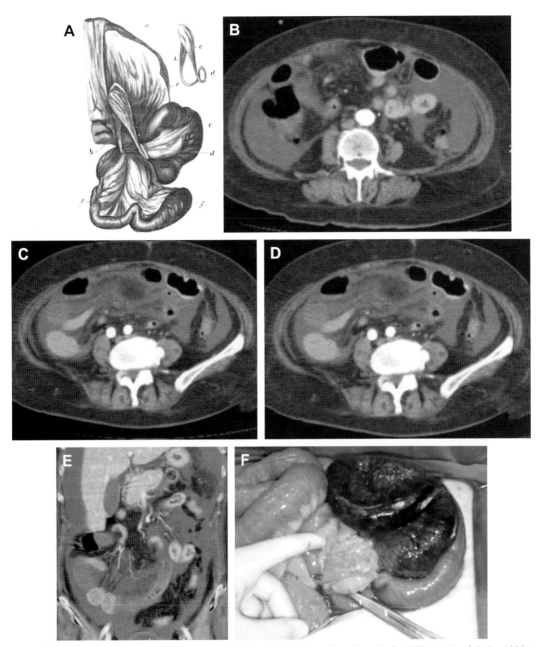

Fig. 18. (A) Strangulation by band. (From Treves F. Intestinal obstruction. New York: William Wood & Co; 1899. p. 37.) MDCT findings in patient with acute abdominal pain and obstructive symptoms: evidence of peritoneal fluid, distension of the intestine predominantly by fluid (B, C), with presence of mesenteric engorgement and parietal thickening of the distended loops (D), some of them characterized by the hyperdense endoluminal content due to hemorrhage, decreased and absence of parietal enhancement of several segment (E). Surgery confirmed the presence of ileal infarction from strangulating band (F).

acute small bowel obstruction; however, most reports describe the usefulness of this imaging method in evaluating the presence, disposition, and degree of air–fluid levels as signs of high-grade obstruction or occlusion.[21–24] The role of sonography as an additional basic imaging method to evaluate the presence of the small bowel is known,[25] especially—but not exclusively—in European countries. Recently, initial experiences on the use of contrast-enhanced ultrasonography in evaluation of bowel ischemia have been described.[26]

The role of CT in diagnosing small bowel obstructions is well known,[27–30] as is its role in detecting the complications and presence of ischemia.[31–46] Most of the report indicated some findings to consider in the evaluation of the ischemia from small bowel occlusion: decreased or absence of bowel wall enhancement, small bowel feces sign, whirl sign, mesenteric edema, mesenteric engorgement, multiple transition point, bowel wall thickening, bowel wall edema, and thin wall. In evaluating a patient with an acute abdominal condition and suspected small bowel occlusion using MDCT, radiologists must evaluate several factors: (1) presence or absence of obstruction, (2) location of the obstruction (small bowel or large bowel), (3) probable cause of the obstruction, (4) degree of the obstruction (simple, complicated), and (5) evidence of ischemic complications or infarct.

The aim of the radiologic report should be to note the presence, cause, and type of obstruction and evaluate its degree.[47] To accomplish a schematic collection of findings related to the disease progression with MDCT, it should theoretically hypothesize a multiple-stage disease progression, from early suspicion to late-stage infarction in small bowel obstruction conditions (Table 1).

Because reaction of the intestine seems to follow the same pathophysiologic progression regardless of the acute injury, at the first stage of the disease, transient spastic reflex ileus and hypotonic ileus could be appreciated in the imaging evaluation. Imaging is performed at onset of acute symptoms because the possibility of finding them is lessened, considering that when a patient comes to the emergency department, he or she already has had the symptoms for several hours. [25,46] The second stage of the disease is more easily appreciated by MDCT because of findings that suggest the presence of an obstruction: various degree of distension of bowel loops by fluid with air–fluid levels and generally no evidence of parietal thickening or decreased wall enhancement (Figs. 9 and 10).

After performing certain medical procedures (eg, nasoenteric tube placement), it should be possible to observe relief of symptoms and obstructive findings or a progression of disease to the occlusive stage. Progression of the disease could produce different patterns, depending on the predominance of the arterial or venous compromise. In closed loop obstructions, the artery and vein are compressed, but because arterial pressure is higher than venous pressure, blood inflow is higher than venous outflow. The consequent appearance of the loop is similar to that of a loop that has impaired mesenteric venous drainage.[36]

At this theoretic third stage of disease, MDCT examination shows an increase in air–fluid distension and thickening of the bowel wall (Fig. 11). If occlusion progresses, the bowel wall becomes more thickened, and vascular engorgement, mesenteric edema, or hemorrhage and endoluminal hemorrhage can be appreciated. These findings, which represent late findings correlated to bowel necrosis, are theoretically considered as the fourth stage of disease (Figs. 12 to 14). The whirl sign, the mesentery peduncle feature, and detection of the transition point and beaks could be helpful in determining the level of the occlusion and the suggestive cause. The status of the intestinal wall should be a crucial point to evaluate, however (Figs. 15 and 16).

Information regarding ischemic complication of the bowel is important for the referring surgeon in order to plan the correct time for a surgical therapy. The surgeon also must consider that the typical patient affected by intestinal obstruction is elderly and often has undergone previous abdominal interventions, so additional, possibly unnecessary surgery could represent a source for future occlusive episodes. Another factor to consider is that if the arterial supply is more tightly compromised from the beginning of the obstruction, the bowel wall might be thin and not enhancing and may show findings similar to those related to not reperfused mesenteric ischemia.[36] MDCT can show evidence of dilated, fluid-filled loops with thin, nonenhancing walls (Figs.16 and 17), which are usually accompanied by mesenteric edema. In this case, searching for the presence of mesentery torsion or transition point could increase the specificity of the diagnosis.

SUMMARY

In acute abdominal conditions, MDCT examination is usually required because of the elevated diagnostic performances of this imaging method in differentiating various types of disease leading to an acute event. Because the intestine is a "dynamic" system, it is incorrect to try to classify the manifestation correlated to the acute injury. A large spectrum of appearances can indicate various diseases, and the same condition can appear in different forms, depending on the "stage" of the disease. Correlation with imaging findings from a previous examination of the patient, knowledge of the patient's clinical history, and laboratory parameters can improve the chances of a correct diagnosis. In the same patient, the acutely ill intestine could present with a different pattern of wall features (Figs. 17 and 18). In the MDCT examination of an acute obstructive syndrome, beyond the evaluation of the morphologic findings of the intestine (eg, dilation, air–fluid level, whirl sign, transition point), which can be well detected with the help of multiplanar reconstructions, it is important to consider the pathophysiology of the bowel wall to better estimate the status of viability, the degree of the obstruction, and the presence of intestinal ischemic complications or infarction.

REFERENCES

1. Treves F. Introduction. In: Intestinal obstructions. New York: William Wood & Co; 1899. p. 1–8.
2. Wangensteen OH. The recognition of obstruction. In: Intestinal obstructions. 2nd edition. Springfield (IL): Charles C. Thomas Publ; 1942. p. 98–116.
3. Treves F. Pathology and morbid anatomy. In: Intestinal obstructions. New York: William Wood & Co; 1899. p. 9–283.
4. Wangensteen OH. The effects of distension. In: Intestinal obstructions. 2nd edition. Springfield (IL): Charles C. Thomas Publ; 1942. p. 8–73.
5. Wangensteen OH. The effects of distension. In: Intestinal obstructions. 3rd edition. Springfield (IL): Charles C. Thomas Publ; 1955. p. 13–96.
6. Ishitani MB, Scott James R. Intestinal obstruction in adults. In: Scott HW, Sawyers JL, editors. Surgery of the stomach, duodenum and small intestine. 2nd edition. Boston: Blackwell Scientific publications; 1992. p. 770–88.
7. Bryk D. The altered colon in colonic obstructions. AJR Am J Roentgenol 1972;115(2):360–7.
8. Frager D, Rovno HD, Baer JW, et al. Prospective evaluation of colonic obstruction with computed tomography. Abdom Imaging 1998;23:141–6.
9. Fisher JK. Abnormal colonic wall thickening on computed tomography. J Comput Assist Tomogr 1983;7:90–7.
10. Simon AM, Birnbaum BA, Jacobs JE. Isolated infarction of the caecum: CT findings in two patients. Radiology 2000;214:513–6.
11. Taourel PG, Deneuville M, Pradel JA, et al. Acute mesenteric ischemia: diagnosis with contrast-enhanced CT. Radiology 1996;199:632–6.
12. Xion L, Chintapalli KN, Dodd GD, et al. Frequency and CT patterns of bowel wall thickening proximal to cancer of the colon. AJR Am J Roentgenol 2004;182:905–9.
13. Frager D. Intestinal obstruction role of CT. Gastroenterol Clin North Am 2002;31(3):777–99.
14. Sinha R, Verma R. Multidetector row computed tomography in bowel obstruction. Part 2. Large bowel obstruction. Clin Radiol 2005;60(10):1068–75.
15. Taourel PG, Garibaldi F, Arrigoni J, et al. Cecal pneumatosis in patients with obstructive colon cancer: correlation of CT findings with bowel viability. AJR Am J Roentgenol 2004;183:1667–71.
16. Taourel P, Kessler N, Lesnik A, et al. Helical CT of large bowel obstruction. Abdom Imaging 2003;28(2):267–75.
17. Kernagis LI, Levine MS, Jacobs GE. Pneumatosis intestinalis in patients with ischemia: correlation of CT findings with viability of bowel. AJR Am J Roentgenol 2003;180:733–6.
18. Wiesner W, MOrtele KJ, Glickman JN, et al. Pneumatosis intestinalis and portomesenteric venous gas in intestinal ischemia: correlation of CT findings with severity of ischemia and clinical outcome. AJR Am J Roentgenol 2001;177:1319–23.
19. Aufort S, Charra L, Lesnik A, et al. Multidetector CT of bowel obstruction: value of post-processing. Eur Radiol 2005;15:2323–9.
20. Khurana B. The whirl sign. Radiology 2003;226(1):69–70.
21. Maglinte DDT, Kelvin FM, Sandrasegaran K, et al. Radiology of small bowel obstruction: contemporary approach and controversies. Abdom Imaging 2005;30(2):160–78.
22. Lappas J, Reyes BL, Maglinte DDT. Abdominal radiography findings in small bowel obstruction: relevance to triage for additional diagnostic imaging. AJR Am J Roentgenol 2001;176:167–74.
23. Thomson WM, Kilani RK, Smith BB, et al. Accuracy of abdominal radiography in acute small bowel obstruction: does reviewers' experience matter? AJR Am J Roentgenol 2007;188:W233–8.
24. Maglinte DDT, Reyes BL, Harmon BH, et al. Reliability and role of plain film radiography and CT in the diagnosis of small bowel obstruction. AJR Am J Roentgenol 1996;167:1451–5.
25. Grassi R, Romano S, D'Amario F, et al. The relevance of free fluid between intestinal loops detected by sonography in the clinical assessment of small bowel obstruction in adults. Eur J Radiol 2004;50(1):5–14.
26. Hata J, Karnada T, Harurna K, et al. Evaluation of bowel ischemia with contrast-enhanced US: initial experience. Radiology 2005;236:712–5.
27. Maglinte DDT, Gage SN, Harmon BH, et al. Obstruction of the small intestine: accuracy and role of CT in diagnosis. Radiology 1993;188:61–4.
28. Lazarus DE, Slywotsky C, Bennett GL, et al. Frequency and relevance of the "small bowel feces" sign on CT in patients with small bowel obstruction. AJR Am J Roentgenol 2004;183:1361–6.
29. Maglinte DDT, Howard TJ, Lillemoe KL, et al. Small bowel obstruction: state of the art imaging and its role in clinical management. Clin Gastroenterol Hepatol 2008;6:130–9.
30. Ros PR, Huprich JE. ACR appropriateness criteria on suspected small bowel obstruction. J Am Coll Radiol 2006;3:838–41.
31. Balthazar EJ, Birnbaum BA, Megibow AJ, et al. Closed loop and strangulating intestinal obstruction: CT signs. Radiology 1992;185:769–75.

32. Ha HK, Kim JS, Lee MS, et al. Differentiation of simple and strangulated small bowel obstructions: usefulness of CT criteria. Radiology 1997;204:507–12.

33. Frager D, Baer JW, Medwind SW, et al. Detection of intestinal ischemia in patients with acute small bowel obstruction due to adhesions or hernia: efficacy of CT. AJR Am J Roentgenol 1996;166:67–71.

34. Vinci R, Angelelli G, Stabile Ianora AA, et al. Vascular complications in intestinal obstructions: the role of computed tomography. Radiol Med (Torino) 1999;98(3):157–61.

35. Makita O, Ikushima I, Matsumoto N, et al. CT differentiation between necrotic and nonnecrotic small bowel in closed loop and strangulating obstruction. Abdom Imaging 1999;24(2):120–4.

36. Chou CK. CT manifestation of bowel ischemia. AJR Am J Roentgenol 2002;178:87–91.

37. Elsayes KM, Menias CO, Smullen TL, et al. Closed-loop small-bowel obstruction: diagnostic patterns by multidetector computed tomography. J Comput Assist Tomogr 2007;31(5):697–701.

38. Sandhu PS, Joe BN, Coakley FV, et al. Bowel transition points: multiplicity and posterior location at CT are associated with small-bowel volvulus. Radiology 2007;245(1):160–7.

39. Sheedy SP, Earnest F 4th, Fletcher JG, et al. CT of small-bowel ischemia associated with obstruction in emergency department patients: diagnostic performance evaluation. Radiology 2006;241(3):729–36.

40. Catel L, Lefèvre F, Lauren V, et al. Occlusion du grele sur bride: quel critère scanographic de gravité rechercher? J Radiol 2003;84(1):27–31 [French].

41. Atri M, McGregor C, McInnes M, et al. Multidetector helical CT in the evaluation of acute small bowel obstruction: comparison of non-enhanced (no oral, rectal or IV contrast) and IV enhanced CT. Eur J Radiol 2008 June 3 [Epub ahead of print].

42. Mallo RD, Salem L, Lalani T, et al. Computed tomography diagnosis of ischemia and complete obstruction in small bowel obstruction: a systematic review. J Gastrointest Surg 2005;9(5):690–4.

43. Sandrasegaran K, Maglinte DD. Imaging of small bowel-related complications following major abdominal surgery. Eur J Radiol 2005;53(3):374–86.

44. Obuz F, Terzi C, Sökmen S, et al. The efficacy of helical CT in the diagnosis of small bowel obstruction. Eur J Radiol 2003;48(3):299–304.

45. Zalcman M, Sy M, Donckier V, et al. Helical CT signs in the diagnosis of intestinal ischemia in small bowel obstruction. AJR Am J Roentgenol 2000;175:1601–7.

46. Grassi R, Di Mizio R, Pinto A, et al. Serial plain abdominal film findings in the assessment of acute abdomen: spastic ileus, hypotonic ileus, mechanical ileus and paralytic ileus. Radiol Med 2004;108(1–2):56–70.

47. Frager D, Medwid SW, Baer WJ, et al. CT of small bowel obstruction: value in establishing the diagnosis and determining the degree and cause. AJR Am J Roentgenol 1994;162(1):37–41.

Differential Diagnosis of Small Bowel Ischemia

Heidi Umphrey, MD, Cheri L. Canon, MD,
Mark E. Lockhart, MD, MPH*

KEYWORDS

- Impaired venous drainage
- Mesenteric arterial hypoperfusion • Thrombosis

Small bowel ischemia, which results from mesenteric arterial hypoperfusion, thrombosis, or impaired venous drainage, is an abdominal emergency. With increasing life expectancy, acute small bowel ischemia represents one of the most serious abdominal conditions in the elderly population.[1–6] Clinical presentation of small bowel ischemia is variable, presenting with a myriad of specific or nonspecific clinical and laboratory findings. The imaging findings of intestinal ischemia have been well reported in the literature but are also nonspecific.[7–9] Therefore, the combination of clinical and imaging data is paramount for definitive and timely diagnosis.

The imaging findings associated with small bowel ischemia (**Fig. 1**) are variable and combinations of findings may be necessary for definitive diagnosis. More specific imaging findings in patients with acute small intestine ischemia include bowel wall gas, mesenteric vessel occlusion, mesenteric venous gas, portal venous gas, or absence of bowel wall enhancement (**Fig. 2**).[7–9] Less specific imaging findings include small bowel wall thickening, mesenteric stranding, and mesenteric fluid.[7–9]

Further complicating the issue, several small intestinal disease processes may mimic ischemia both clinically and radiographically. These alternate diagnoses include infectious, inflammatory, and infiltrative processes. In this review, we discuss the differential diagnosis for small bowel ischemia.

INFECTION
Mycobacterium Avium-Intracellulare

Systemic infection with *Mycobacterium avium-intracellulare* affects multiple organs and has been called pseudo-Whipple disease because of clinical, histologic, and radiologic similarities.[10] These patients are immunocompromised and usually present with watery diarrhea and malabsorption. Clinically, the chronicity of disease may help differentiate it from small bowel ischemia, which is characterized by acute symptoms.

CT findings include thickened small bowel more pronounced in the jejunum, hepatomegaly, and splenomegaly.[11] Focal, low-density lesions are often present in the spleen. Such lesions are not seen in Whipple disease. Bulky mesenteric and retroperitoneal adenopathy is frequently seen in disseminated *M avium-intracellulare* infection and should be differentiated from lymphoma.[12] Low-density adenopathy associated with disseminated *M avium-intracellulare* may provide a clue to the diagnosis, but this appearance is more frequently seen in disseminated mycobacterium tuberculosis infection (**Fig. 3**).[11]

Cytomegalovirus

Cytomegalovirus is a member of the herpes virus group and is transmitted by blood transfusion or through sexual contact. The virus usually remains dormant in the normal host but can be reactivated if the patient becomes immunosuppressed. In active infection, mucosal ulcerations are typical within the small bowel, resulting in hemorrhagic enteritis.[13–15]

CT findings include nonspecific mural thickening. Barium studies also show areas of subtle narrowing and mucosal ulceration (**Fig. 4**).[13] However, definitive diagnosis may require biopsy with immunohistochemical stains to confirm.

Department of Radiology, JTN358, University of Alabama at Birmingham, 619 19th Street South, Birmingham, AL 35249-6830, USA
* Corresponding author.
E-mail address: mlockhart@uabmc.edu (M.E. Lockhart).

Radiol Clin N Am 46 (2008) 943–952
doi:10.1016/j.rcl.2008.06.004

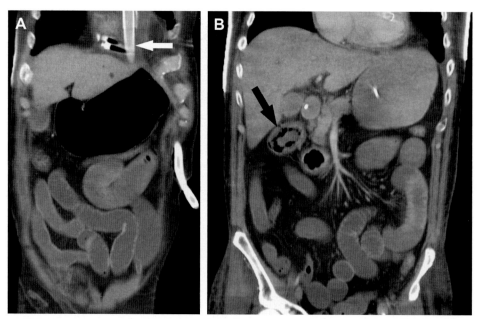

Fig. 1. Global ischemia. (*A*) Coronal image from contrast-enhanced CT reveals diffusely dilated small bowel with mild mural thickening in a patient with cardiomyopathy and profound hypotensive episode who subsequently underwent placement of a left ventricular assist device (*arrow*). (*B*) Pneumatosis is present in the hepatic flexure of the colon (*arrow*). Exploratory laparotomy revealed diffuse ischemia of the majority of the gut. Patient subsequently died.

Cryptosporidiosis

Cryptosporidium is a gastrointestinal parasite that results in diffuse watery diarrhea in patients with AIDS.[16] CT findings demonstrate wall thickening more often involving the proximal small bowel loops and stomach.[17] The CT appearance is similar to that of giardiasis, *M avium-intracellulare*, Zollinger-Ellison syndrome, early ischemic bowel, and eosinophilic gastroenteritis. Clinical history is important in establishing a diagnosis. However, definitive diagnosis often relies on special stains of stool samples.

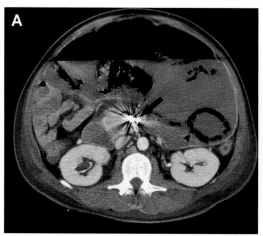
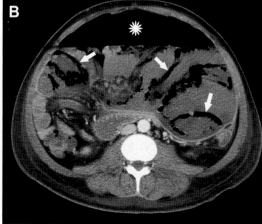

Fig. 2. Ischemia with liquefactive necrosis. (*A*) CT image through the upper abdomen reveals vascular coils in the superior mesenteric artery (*arrow*). Coils were placed for life-threatening pseudoaneurysm hemorrhage secondary to pancreatitis. (*B*) Extensive small bowel pneumatosis (*arrows*) with dilatation, pneumoperitoneum (*asterisk*), and free fluid. Exploratory laparotomy revealed diffuse necrosis too extensive for resection. Patient subsequently died in hospice care.

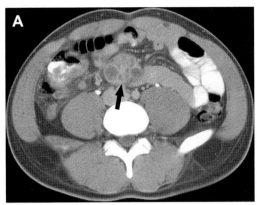
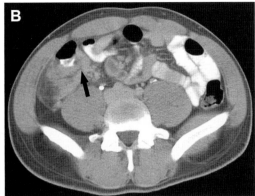

Fig. 3. Tuberculous ileocolitis. Contrast-enhanced CT in this 28-year-old nursing student from Tanzania reveals (*A*) low-density mesenteric lymphadenopathy (*arrow*) and (*B*) marked thickening of the terminal ileum and colon (*arrow*).

Giardiasis

Giardia lamblia is a multiflagellate protozoan that was once thought to be a harmless commensal organism. However, despite its variable clinical presentation, it is now known to cause severe diarrhea and malabsorption.[18,19] The organism tends to inhabit the duodenum and jejunum.[20]

Imaging findings consist of mural thickening, increased luminal secretions, and disordered motility.[21,22] The finding of contrast flocculations may be helpful in differentiating this entity from bowel ischemia. The diagnosis of *G lamblia* is most often accomplished by identification of the characteristic cysts in the stool or tissue biopsy with identification of organisms.

Whipple Disease

Whipple disease is a chronic multisystemic condition that affects adults and is caused by gram-positive bacilli.[23] Histologically, there is characteristic infiltration of the small bowel mucosa and submucosa with foamy macrophages that contain periodic acid-Schiff–positive glycoprotein granules.[24] Clinical presentation includes a malabsorption syndrome and chronic diarrhea.

CT findings include thickening of the small bowel folds more commonly involving the jejunum, without bowel dilation or abnormal transit time.[24] Bulky, fat-density mesenteric and retroperitoneal lymph are characteristic and suggest diagnosis.[25,26] The additional findings of hepatosplenomegaly and ascites may also be helpful in establishing the specific diagnosis.[25,26]

INFLAMMATORY DISEASE
Crohn Disease

Crohn disease is a transmural inflammatory bowel disease that can involve the small bowel, particularly the terminal ileum. Crohn disease may cause continuous involvement or skip areas within the bowel wall.

The most characteristic small bowel finding of Crohn disease by CT is the presence of wall thickening, particularly involving the terminal ileum (**Fig. 5**). As the disease progresses, the wall can measure greater than 1 cm in thickness and there may be associated adjacent mesenteric stranding.[27] Wall thickening is usually symmetric and homogeneous but can be eccentric. Extensive wall thickening associated with luminal narrowing that persists over time may indicate the presence of stricture. Occasionally, the wall may have an intermediate layer of low density known as a "double

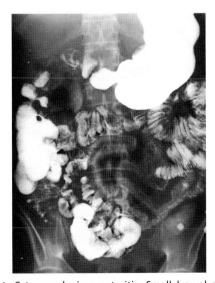

Fig. 4. Cytomegalovirus enteritis. Small bowel series image shows mural thickening of small bowel loops with luminal narrowing.

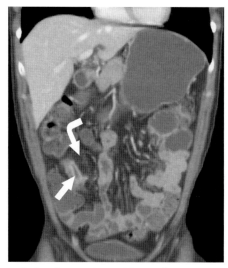

Fig. 5. Crohn disease. Coronal image from CT enterography performed in a 47-year-old woman with Crohn disease reveals terminal ileal mural thickening with mucosal hyperenhancement (*straight arrow*), the most sensitive finding for active disease. Note engorged vasa recta (*curved arrow*).

fat is easily identified, and there may be prominence of the vasa recta, known as the "comb sign" (see **Fig. 5**), due to hyperemia of the bowel segment. These findings would not be expected in mesenteric ischemia. Complications of Crohn disease include intra-abdominal abscesses, fistula, and strictures. These are well evaluated with CT and can be useful in establishing a definitive diagnosis.[30]

Celiac Disease

Celiac disease stems from sensitivity to gluten products. This sensitivity leads to villous atrophy of the small bowel. Patients usually present with diarrhea or weight loss but can present with abdominal pain. Imaging findings may include small bowel dilation, a reversal of the normal jejunoileal fold pattern (**Fig. 6**), fold separation, and nonobstructing small bowel intussusception.[31,32] Extraintestinal manifestations, such as lymphadenopathy, can be seen. Definitive diagnosis requires mucosal biopsy demonstrating villous atrophy.

halo" or "halo," which represents submucosal edema or fatty deposition.[28,29] The halo sign is not seen in neoplastic disease of the small bowel but may be present in a variety of inflammatory conditions, such as radiation enteritis, graft-versus-host disease, and chronic ischemic bowel. Another characteristic finding of Crohn disease is fibrofatty proliferation that can displace bowel, simulating a mass or abscess on abdominal radiographs or barium studies.[27] On CT, the prominent

Small Bowel Diverticulitis

The frequency of acquired diverticula detectable by imaging in the small bowel is reportedly 2.3%.[33] Small bowel diverticula can either be congenital (containing all three layers of bowel wall) or acquired.[34] Acquired small bowel diverticula are a result of acquired mucosal herniation through the muscular wall and are more common in the jejunum than the ileum.

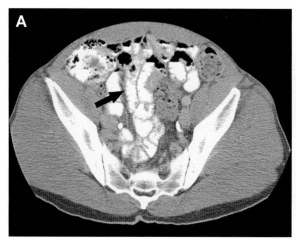
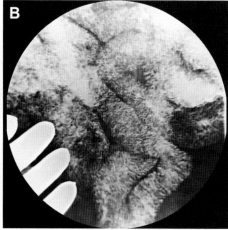

Fig. 6. Sprue. (*A*) Contrast-enhanced CT image through the pelvis reveals, in this patient with sprue, increased number of folds in the distal ileum (*arrow*), a process called "jejunization" of the ileum. Jejunization can be confused with mural thickening, particularly if the lumen is collapsed and there is poor oral contrast delineation of the folds. (*B*) Contrast fluoroscopy confirms increased fold pattern.

On CT, diverticula appear as outpouchings from the bowel lumen that contain air or contrast material and can be difficult to differentiate from overlapping loops of small bowel. Acute complications of the small bowel diverticula occur in 7% to 10% of patients and include perforation (**Fig. 7**), intestinal obstruction, hemorrhage, and diverticulitis.[35] CT findings of small bowel diverticulitis include an inflammatory mass or regional stranding of the adjacent fat localized to small bowel with adjacent mesenteric edema.[36] Hyperemia and widely patent appearance of the mesenteric vessels help differentiate this diagnosis from ischemia.

Radiation Enteritis

Radiation enteritis, one possible complication of abdominal radiotherapy, results from ischemic and subsequent fibrotic injury to the small bowel mucosa and submucosa secondary to obliterative arteritis. The distal small bowel is most commonly affected. Clinical symptoms include nausea, vomiting, and abdominal pain. The frequency and severity of radiation enteritis depend on the radiation dose received, treatment volume, and fractionation scale. When doses of 5000 rad were used over a 6-week period, the incidence of small bowel complications requiring surgery was reported to be as high as 10% in one study.[37]

The CT appearance of acute radiation enteritis consists of small bowel wall thickening, edema, and inflammatory changes in adjacent mesenteric fat. A submucosal halo within the bowel wall can be seen representing edema or inflammation. However, the appearance differs from that seen in Crohn disease, as the halo is not symmetric.[38] Chronic radiation changes can also occur 1 to 2 years after the completion of radiation therapy and are characterized on CT by fixed thickened small bowel loops, stenoses, or fistulas. Increased density in the mesentery with stranding is also a common finding. Clinical history and knowledge of radiation ports are important in establishing a diagnosis to differentiate radiation enteritis from small bowel ischemia.

Graft-Versus-Host Disease

Graft-versus-host disease is a life-threatening complication of allogeneic bone marrow transplantation. It is thought to occur when donor lymphocytes of the graft mount an immune response against the host. This process occurs usually between 10 and 50 days after transplantation. The small bowel can be affected, resulting in a clinical presentation of abdominal cramps and diarrhea.

Findings on imaging include small bowel fold thickening, resulting in luminal narrowing (**Fig. 8**).[39] If severe, the bowel folds may be effaced, resulting in a featureless, tubular appearance.[39,40] Prolonged contrast-agent coating of the intestine has been reported in cases of severe mucosal disease where the barium can actually become incorporated into the bowel wall as mucosal ulcerations heal.[41,42] Additionally, CT may show a halo of decreased attenuation within the wall as well as adjacent inflammatory changes in mesentery.[39] The morphologic abnormalities may be diffuse or segmental and are often accompanied by excess intraluminal fluid and rapid bowel transit time. The length of small bowel involvement in graft-versus-host disease is more extensive than in Crohn disease or radiation enteritis. However, the most helpful finding in determining

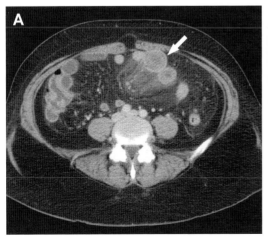
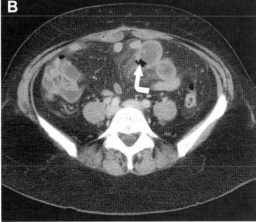

Fig. 7. Perforated jejunal diverticulum. (*A*) Contrast-enhanced CT in a 58-year-old man with abdominal pain reveals focal small bowel thickening and edema (*arrow*). (*B*) Focal collection of extraluminal gas (*curved arrow*).

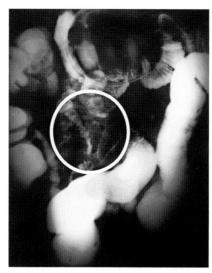

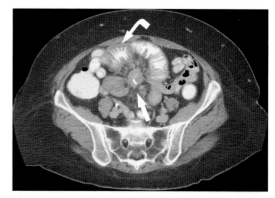

Fig. 9. Carcinoid. Contrast-enhanced CT in a 59-year-old woman reveals spiculated, calcified mesenteric nodal mass (*straight arrow*) with mural thickening (*curved arrow*) of contiguous small bowel loops.

Fig. 8. Graft-versus-host disease. Enteroclysis shows rapid transit of contrast to the colon. Transit took less than 10 minutes. Severe mural thickening of small bowel loops (*circle*).

the diagnosis is clinical history. Definitive diagnosis may require tissue biopsy.

Neoplasm and Infiltrative Disease

Small bowel malignancy

Tumor involvement of the small bowel may be primary or metastatic in nature. Primary small bowel malignancies are relatively rare.[43] Carcinoid tumor is the most common type.[44] This tumor arises from neuroendocrine cells of the submucosa, usually in the distal ileum, where there is the highest concentration of these cells. The primary tumor, often so small that it goes unseen, presents as a calcified, spiculated mesenteric metastatic nodal mass (**Fig. 9**). Because the mass obstructs venous and lymphatic drainage and secretes vasoactive amines, adjacent small bowel loops are usually thickened. The presence of a mesenteric mass and a tethered appearance of the small bowel loops help differentiate small bowel malignancies from ischemia.

Most lymphoma of the small bowel is non-Hodgkin type and has a protean appearance.[43] Aneurysmal dilatation with mural thickening (**Fig. 10**) is pathognomonic for small bowel lymphoma. Obstructing strictures are uncommon in lymphoma. Primary adenocarcinoma usually occurs in the duodenum or jejunum (**Fig. 11**). In addition to a focal mass, primary adenocarcinoma can present with circumferential wall thickening but affects a shorter segment than does ischemia.

Metastases to the small bowel are often hematogenous from bronchogenic or breast carcinoma

and melanoma. These lesions are usually polypoid and eccentric, thus making them readily distinguishable from ischemia. Peritoneal metastases from ovarian or colon carcinoma can present with circumferential thickening. However, there are typically other findings of peritoneal carcinomatosis.

Amyloidosis

In cases of generalized amyloidosis, the small bowel is involved more frequently than any other portion of the gastrointestinal tract.[45,46] Amyloid is deposited around small blood vessels in the submucosa and between fibers within the muscular layers of the bowel wall. Definitive diagnosis requires histologic identification of the amyloid in affected tissues. Rectal biopsy has been used in the past to diagnose systemic amyloidosis.[45]

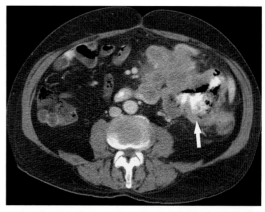

Fig. 10. Lymphoma. Contrast-enhanced CT reveals excavated, aneurysmal dilatation of thickened loop of small bowel (*arrow*) in patient with non-Hodgkin lymphoma.

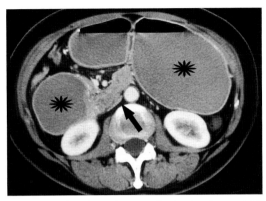

Fig. 11. Duodenal carcinoma. Contrast-enhanced CT shows severe dilatation of stomach and proximal duodenum (*asterisks*) to the level of a heterogenous duodenal mass (*arrow*).

Small bowel studies reveal decreased motility and normal intestinal secretion.[47] CT findings include bowel wall thickening, dilatation, and mesenteric infiltration.[47,48] Adenopathy or amyloid infiltration of other organs may be present and can assist in the differential diagnosis. In amyloidosis, adenopathy has greater density and less bulk than that seen in Whipple disease.

OTHER ETIOLOGIES IN THE DIFFERENTIAL DIAGNOSIS
Scleroderma

Systemic scleroderma is a generalized disorder of small arteries, microvessels, and connective tissue of unknown origin. Involvement of the small bowel can occur. Narrowed intervalvular distance disproportionate for the degree of dilation, described as "hide-bound" small bowel, is characteristic of scleroderma of the small bowel (Fig. 12).[49]

Lymphangiectasia

Intestinal lymphangiectasia is a rare entity that presents with severe edema, protein-losing enteropathy, ascites, and pleural effusions.[50] Pathologically, there is dilatation of the lymphatics within the mesentery and within the mucosa and submucosa of the small bowel. The condition may be primary, resulting from a congenital lymphatic blockage, or secondary, resulting from inflammatory or neoplastic involvement of lymphatics.[51]

CT findings include diffuse small bowel wall thickening, which is a result of engorgement of villi containing the dilated lymphatics.[52] Also, according to one report, the halo sign has been seen in a patient with primary intestinal lymphangiectasia.[53]

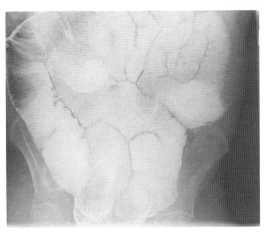

Fig. 12. Scleroderma. Contrast fluoroscopy of the small bowel in this 40-year-old man with polymyositis and scleroderma reveals diffuse dilatation with dilution of the barium from large quantities of retained fluid. Note closely spaced small bowel folds, "hide-bound," resulting from selective fibrosis of the inner circular layer of the muscularis propria. Outer longitudinal layer normally contracts, foreshortening the bowel with resultant increased fold density despite luminal dilatation.

Intramural Hemorrhage

Among the many causes of intestinal hemorrhage are ischemia, trauma, vasculitis, coagulopathies, and anticoagulation therapy.[54] Bleeding usually occurs within the submucosal layer. The CT appearance of regular fold thickening is known as the "picket fence" appearance on contrast fluoroscopic examination. This may be diffuse or segmental, depending on the etiology of the hemorrhage. Bleeding tracks along the submucosal compartment and can present on CT as an intramural mass that narrows the lumen of the bowel and could be confused with a small bowel tumor.[55] If the hemorrhage is acute, the hematoma may have high density on noncontrast CT images. Intramural hemorrhage usually involves a short segment less than 15 cm as opposed to small bowel ischemia, which involves a segment of intestine usually longer than 30 cm.[56] Also, CT findings reveal a wall thickness of 1 cm or more in small bowel wall hemorrhage (Fig. 13), and less than 1 cm in intestinal ischemia.[56] Mesenteric fluid or hemoperitoneum are often associated with bowel wall hemorrhage or injury.[57,58]

Angioedema

Angioedema is a process by which capillaries leak serum. There are several etiologies, including angiotensin-converting enzyme (ACE) inhibitors (Fig. 14), hereditary factors, and allergic

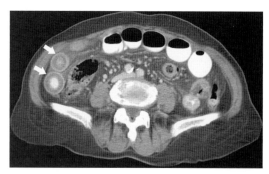

Fig. 13. Hemorrhage. Contrast-enhanced CT in an 81-year-old woman with chronic anticoagulation for deep venous thrombosis and acute abdominal pain reveals circumferential, smooth thickening (*arrows*) of a short segment of small bowel. Note marked degree of thickening without luminal distension, as well as adjacent mesenteric fluid.

reactions.[59–61] ACE-inhibitor edema does not always occur during the initial period of taking this medication. In fact, it has been documented to occur 9 years after the onset of enalapril therapy.[62] When ACE-inhibitors are the etiology, resolution of findings can be seen within 24 hours of drug cessation. The findings on CT are nonspecific but may reveal bowel wall thickening with fluid density, also known as the "halo" sign.[63]

Pneumatosis Intestinalis

Pneumatosis intestinalis is the presence of gas within the bowel wall. It can be secondary to a variety of etiologies, both benign and life-threatening.[64–67] Depending upon the etiology,

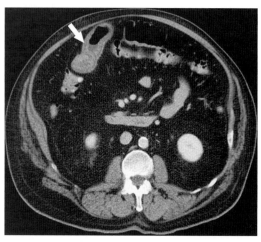

Fig. 14. Angioedema. Contrast-enhanced CT in a 63-year-old man with acute onset of abdominal pain and history of taking ACE-inhibitor reveals short-segment mural thickening (*arrow*) with low-density mural edema.

pneumatosis intestinalis can be asymptomatic or present with an acute abdomen. Correlation with serum lactate acid levels is the most helpful means in identifying "benign" versus "malignant" pneumatosis. In fact, pneumatosis intestinalis associated with a lactic acid level of greater than 2 mmol/L has been associated with greater than 80% mortality.[68] This presence of gas in the small bowel wall can be seen on abdominal radiographs. However, CT is more sensitive (see **Figs. 1** and **2**).

SUMMARY

The differential diagnosis of small bowel ischemia is vast, and many small bowel pathologies have similar imaging findings. Careful correlation of clinical data and specific CT findings is imperative to identify the correct diagnosis.

ACKNOWLEDGMENTS

The authors would like to thank Trish Thurman, for her help in manuscript preparation, and Anthony Zagar, for his photography assistance.

REFERENCES

1. Brandt L, Boley S, Goldberg L, et al. Colitis in the elderly. A reappraisal. Am J Gastroenterol 1981; 76(3):239–45.
2. Ruotolo RA, Evans SR. Mesenteric ischemia in the elderly. Clin Geriatr Med 1999;15(3):527–57.
3. Levine JS, Jacobson ED. Intestinal ischemic disorders. Dig Dis 1995;13(1):3–24.
4. Inderbitzi R, Wagner HE, Seiler C, et al. Acute mesenteric ischaemia. Eur J Surg 1992;158(2):123–6.
5. Vinen O Jr, Laurikka J, Salenius JP, et al. Acute intestinal ischaemia. A review of 214 cases. Ann Chir Gynaecol 1994;83(1):22–5.
6. Duron JJ, Montcel ST, Berger A, et al. Prevalence and risk factors of mortality and morbidity after operation for adhesive postoperative small bowel obstruction. Am J Surg 2008;195(6):726–34.
7. Yamada K, Saeki M, Yamaguchi T, et al. Acute mesenteric ischemia. CT and plain radiographic analysis of 26 cases. Clin Imaging 1998;22(1):34–41.
8. Alpern MB, Glazer GM, Francis IR. Ischemic or infarcted bowel: CT findings. Radiology 1988; 166(1 Pt 1):149–52.
9. Klein HM, Lensing R, Klosterhalfen B, et al. Diagnostic imaging of mesenteric infarction. Radiology 1995; 197(1):79–82.
10. Poorman JC, Katon RM. Small bowel involvement by Mycobacterium avium complex in a patient with AIDS: endoscopic, histologic, and radiographic similarities to Whipple's disease. Gastrointest Endosc 1994;40(6):753–9.

11. Radin DR. Intraabdominal mycobacterium tuberculosis vs mycobacterium avium-intracellulare infections in patients with AIDS: distinction based on CT findings. AJR Am J Roentgenol 1991;156(3):487–91.

12. Nyberg DA, Federle MP, Jeffrey RB, et al. Abdominal CT findings of disseminated Mycobacterium avium-intracellulare in AIDS. AJR Am J Roentgenol 1985; 145(2):297–9.

13. Teixidor HS, Honig CL, Norsoph E, et al. Cytomegalovirus infection of the alimentary canal: radiologic findings with pathologic correlation. Radiology 1987;163(2):317–23.

14. Sugimoto T, Soumura M, Kawasaki M, et al. Cytomegalovirus-induced small-bowel hemorrhage in a patient with nonsystemic vasculitic neuropathy. Clin Rheumatol 2006;25(4):575–6.

15. Ryu KH, Yi SY. Cytomegalovirus ileitis in an immunocompetent elderly adult. World J Gastroenterol 2006;12(31):5084–6.

16. Lumadue JA, Manabe YC, Moore RD, et al. A clinicopathologic analysis of AIDS-related cryptosporidiosis. AIDS 1998;12(18):2459–66.

17. Berk RN, Wall SD, McArdle CB, et al. Cryptosporidiosis of the stomach and small intestine in patients with AIDS. AJR Am J Roentgenol 1984;143(3): 549–54.

18. Moore GT, Cross WM, McGuire D, et al. Epidemic giardiasis at a ski resort. N Engl J Med 1969; 281(8):402–7.

19. Yardley JH, Bayless TM. Giardiasis. Gastroenterology 1967;52(2):301–4.

20. Morecki R, Parker JG. Ultrastructural studies of the human Giardia lamblia and subjacent jejunal mucosa in a subject with steatorrhea. Gastroenterology 1967; 52(2):151–64.

21. Marshak RH, Ruoff M, Lindner AE. Roentgen manifestations of Giardiasis. Am J Roentgenol Radium Ther Nucl Med 1968;104(3):557–60.

22. Peterson GM. Intestinal changes in giardia lamblia infestation. Am J Roentgenol Radium Ther Nucl Med 1957;77(4):670–7.

23. Cohen AS, Schimmel EM, Holt PR, et al. Ultrastructural abnormalities in Whipple's disease. Proc Soc Exp Biol Med 1960;105:411–4.

24. Fleming JL, Wiesner RH, Shorter RG. Whipple's disease: clinical, biochemical, and histopathologic features and assessment of treatment in 29 patients. Mayo Clin Proc 1988;63(6):539–51.

25. Rijke AM, Falke TH, de Vries RR. Computed tomography in Whipple disease. J Comput Assist Tomogr 1983;7(6):1101–2.

26. Li DK, Rennie CS. Abdominal computed tomography in Whipple's disease. J Comput Assist Tomogr 1981; 5(2):249–52.

27. Gore RM, Marn CS, Kirby DF, et al. CT findings in ulcerative, granulomatous, and indeterminate colitis. AJR Am J Roentgenol 1984;143(2):279–84.

28. Frager DH, Goldman M, Beneventano TC. Computed tomography in Crohn disease. J Comput Assist Tomogr 1983;7(5):819–24.

29. Jones B, Fishman EK, Hamilton SR, et al. Submucosal accumulation of fat in inflammatory bowel disease: CT/pathologic correlation. J Comput Assist Tomogr 1986;10(5):759–63.

30. Fishman EK, Wolf EJ, Jones B, et al. CT evaluation of Crohn's disease: effect on patient management. AJR Am J Roentgenol 1987;148(3):537–40.

31. Rubesin SE, Herlinger H, Saul SH, et al. Adult celiac disease and its complications. Radiographics 1989; 9(6):1045–66.

32. Strobl PW, Warshauer DM. CT diagnosis of celiac disease. J Comput Assist Tomogr 1995;19(2):319–20.

33. Maglinte DD, Chernish SM, DeWeese R, et al. Acquired jejunoileal diverticular disease: subject review. Radiology 1986;158(3):577–80.

34. Caplan LH, Jacobson HG. Small intestinal diverticulosis. Am J Roentgenol Radium Ther Nucl Med 1964;92:1048–60.

35. Roses DF, Gouge TH, Scher KS, et al. Perforated diverticula of the jejunum and ileum. Am J Surg 1976;132(5):649–52.

36. Greenstein S, Jones B, Fishman EK, et al. Small-bowel diverticulitis: CT findings. AJR Am J Roentgenol 1986;147(2):271–4.

37. Romsdahl MM, Withers HR. Radiotherapy combined with curative surgery. Its use as therapy for carcinoma of the sigmoid colon and rectum. Arch Surg 1978;113(4):446–53.

38. Fishman EK, Zinreich ES, Jones B, et al. Computed tomographic diagnosis of radiation ileitis. Gastrointest Radiol 1984;9(2):149–52.

39. Jones B, Fishman EK, Kramer SS, et al. Computed tomography of gastrointestinal inflammation after bone marrow transplantation. AJR Am J Roentgenol 1986;146(4):691–5.

40. Jones B, Kramer SS, Saral R, et al. Gastrointestinal inflammation after bone marrow transplantation: graft-versus-host disease or opportunistic infection? AJR Am J Roentgenol 1988;150(2):277–81.

41. Ma LD, Jones B, Lazenby AJ, et al. Persistent oral contrast agent lining the intestine in severe mucosal disease: elucidation of radiographic appearance. Radiology 1994;191(3):747–9.

42. Fisk JD, Shulman HM, Greening RR, et al. Gastrointestinal radiographic features of human graft-vs.-host disease. AJR Am J Roentgenol 1981; 136(2):329–36.

43. Horton KM, Fishman EK. Multidetector-row computed tomography and 3-dimensional computed tomography imaging of small bowel neoplasms: current concept in diagnosis. J Comput Assist Tomogr 2004;28(1):106–16.

44. Hatzaras I, Palesty JA, Abir F, et al. Small-bowel tumors: epidemiologic and clinical characteristics

of 1260 cases from the Connecticut tumor registry. Arch Surg 2007;142(3):229–35.

45. Tada S, Iida M, Yao T, et al. Gastrointestinal amyloidosis: radiologic features by chemical types. Radiology 1994;190(1):37–42.

46. Gilat T, Revach M, Sohar E. Deposition of amyloid in the gastrointestinal tract. Gut 1969;10(2): 98–104.

47. Kala Z, Valek V, Kysela P. Amyloidosis of the small intestine. Eur J Radiol 2007;63(1):105–9.

48. Kim SH, Han JK, Lee KH, et al. Abdominal amyloidosis: spectrum of radiological findings. Clin Radiol 2003;58(8):610–20.

49. Horowitz AL, Meyers MA. The "hide-bound" small bowel of scleroderma: characteristic mucosal fold pattern. AJR Am J Roentgenol Radium Ther Nucl Med 1973;119(2):332–4.

50. Shimkin PM, Waldmann TA, Krugman RL. Intestinal lymphangiectasia. Am J Roentgenol Radium Ther Nucl Med 1970;110(4):827–41.

51. Fox U, Lucani G. Disorders of the intestinal mesenteric lymphatic system. Lymphology 1993;26(2): 61–6.

52. Fakhri A, Fishman EK, Jones B, et al. Primary intestinal lymphangiectasia: clinical and CT findings. J Comput Assist Tomogr 1985;9(4):767–70.

53. Stevens RL, Jones B, Fishman EK. The CT halo sign: a new finding in intestinal lymphangiectasia. J Comput Assist Tomogr 1997;21(6):1005–7.

54. Bartnicke BJ, Balfe DM. CT appearance of intestinal ischemia and intramural hemorrhage. Radiol Clin North Am 1994;32(5):845–60.

55. Roberts JL, Dalen K, Bosanko CM, et al. CT in abdominal and pelvic trauma. Radiographics 1993; 13(4):735–52.

56. Macari M, Chandarana H, Balthazar E, et al. Intestinal ischemia versus intramural hemorrhage: CT evaluation. AJR Am J Roentgenol 2003;180(1): 177–84.

57. Levine CD, Gonzales RN, Wachsberg RH, et al. CT findings of bowel and mesenteric injury. J Comput Assist Tomogr 1997;21(6):974–9.

58. Cook DE, Walsh JW, Vick CW, et al. Upper abdominal trauma: pitfalls in CT diagnosis. Radiology 1986; 159(1):65–9.

59. Abdelmalek MF, Douglas DD. Lisinopril-induced isolated visceral angioedema: review of ACE-inhibitor–induced small bowel angioedema. Dig Dis Sci 1997;42(4):847–50.

60. Pearson KD, Buchignani JS, Shimkin PM, et al. Hereditary angioneurotic edema of the gastrointestinal tract. Am J Roentgenol Radium Ther Nucl Med 1972; 116(2):256–61.

61. Polger M, Kuhlman JE, Hansen FC 3rd, et al. Computed tomography of angioedema of small bowel due to reaction to radiographic contrast medium. J Comput Assist Tomogr 1988;12(6):1044–6.

62. Orr KK, Myers JR. Intermittent visceral edema induced by long-term enalapril administration. Ann Pharmacother 2004;38(5):825–7.

63. De Backer AI, De Schepper AM, Vandevenne JE, et al. CT of angioedema of the small bowel. AJR Am J Roentgenol 2001;176(3):649–52.

64. Keene JG. Pneumatosis cystoides intestinalis and intramural intestinal gas. J Emerg Med 1989;7(6): 645–50.

65. Knechtle SJ, Davidoff AM, Rice RP. Pneumatosis intestinalis. Surgical management and clinical outcome. Ann Surg 1990;212(2):160–5.

66. Heng Y, Schuffler MD, Haggitt RC, et al. Pneumatosis intestinalis: a review. Am J Gastroenterol 1995;90(10): 1747–58.

67. Pear BL. Pneumatosis intestinalis: a review. Radiology 1998;207(1):13–9.

68. Hawn MT, Canon CL, Lockhart ME, et al. Serum lactic acid determines the outcomes of CT diagnosis of pneumatosis of the gastrointestinal tract. Am Surg 2004;70(1):19–23.

Index

Note: Page numbers of article titles are in **boldface** type.

Radiol Clin N Am 46 (2008) 953–956
doi:10.1016/S0033-8389(08)00169-3
0033-8389/08/$ – see front matter © 2008 Elsevier Inc. All rights reserved.

Moving?

Make sure your subscription moves with you!

To notify us of your new address, find your **Clinics Account Number** (located on your mailing label above your name), and contact customer service at:

E-mail: elspcs@elsevier.com

800-654-2452 (subscribers in the U.S. & Canada)
1-407-563-6020 (subscribers outside of the U.S. & Canada)

Fax number: 407-363-9661

Elsevier Periodicals Customer Service
6277 Sea Harbor Drive
Orlando, FL 32887-4800

*To ensure uninterrupted delivery of your subscription, please notify us at least 4 weeks in advance of move.